chronic

a memoir
of illness
and healing

REBECCA DIMYAN

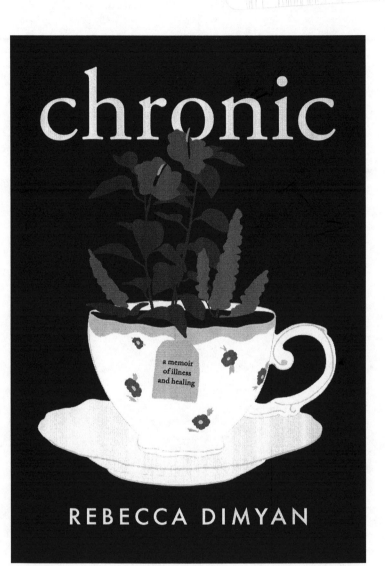

chronic

a memoir

REBECCA DIMYAN

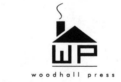

Woodhall Press | Norwalk, CT

Woodhall Press, 81 Old Saugatuck Road, Norwalk, CT 06855
WoodhallPress.com

Cover design: Danny Sancho
Layout artist: L.J. Mucci

Library of Congress Cataloging-in-Publication Data available

ISBN 978-1-954907-11-9   (paper: alk paper)
ISBN 978-1-954907-12-6   (electronic)

First Edition
Distributed by Independent Publishers Group
(800) 888-4741

Printed in the United States of America

This is a work of creative nonfiction. All of the events in this memoir are true to
the best of the author's memory. Some names and identifying features have been
changed to protect the identity of certain parties. The author in no way represents
any company, corporation, or brand, mentioned herein. The views expressed in
this memoir are solely those of the author.

To anyone who has ever known pain & everyone who has ever needed hope

Excerpts of this book have previously been published in:

The Mighty
Endometriosis News
HelloGiggles

Author's Note

Let me begin with a confession: I never wanted to write this book. This memoir is a collection of secrets I never planned to share, the advice I never felt qualified to give, and the hope I never expected to find. In it, I explore emotions and events and very intimate details of my life that are excruciating and I was initially uncomfortable with these stories appearing in print. However, as I began writing short pieces about my chronic illness and the practices I found helpful in managing it, many women reached out to me. They shared their stories, experiences, frustrations, and feelings of utter helplessness— all emotions I had also endured. Some asked for guidance. Others simply thanked me for letting them know that they weren't alone. These messages, these women are the reason I wrote this book.

But what makes me qualified to share my experience? My pain has improved drastically since turning to alternative treatments, but does that mean I am still chronically ill? Can I share my story as if I am an expert in pain if I don't feel this way on a daily basis anymore? The answer, I believe, is yes. I still have bad pain days sometimes. There is no definitive cure for endometriosis; however, I believe there is a better way to manage it than what Western medicine suggests. Eastern Medicine has given me my life back. I do not claim to be any kind of medical professional; I am simply a woman, a writer, a teacher, a daughter, a mother, and an endo warrior. And this is my story.

Pain is trauma. Being vulnerable in memoir is terrifying. Will you think less of me when I disclose my first experience of pelvic pain? Will that change your opinion of me, and therefore, your willingness to hear my story and consider my advice? We spend so much time now attacking each other, not listening to those with differing views, opinions, and experiences. Will you dislike me or judge me because I made mistakes along the way? Because I follow a non-traditional path? Am I too different, too imperfect, too cured, not cured enough?

One could argue that we've come a long way from diagnoses of hysteria and proscriptions of confinement in asylums for treatment of women in pain, but have we really? While we may not lock women up for experiencing chronic illness anymore, in 2022, her pain is often dismissed or normalized—oftentimes by medical professionals.

One in ten women suffer from endometriosis. That's approximately 176 million women worldwide.[1] On average, it takes a woman five to seven years to get a diagnosis. The seemingly infinite cycle of diagnosis and misdiagnosis is like a broken carousel you can't get off. Most women will undergo surgery multiple times with some ultimately removing organs altogether. Endo is regarded as the most aggressive and painful disease a woman can experience outside of cancer. This chronic illness causes tissue similar to the tissue that lines the uterus to grow on other organs such as the ovaries, fallopian tubes, and pelvis. In some cases, the abnormal tissue can also grow on other organs like

---

1   Endometriosis.org. *Facts about Endometriosis – Endometriosis.org*, http://endometriosis.org/resources/articles/facts-about-endometriosis/

the bowel, kidneys, and even lungs. Endometriosis can cause pain, inflammation, irregular periods, and sometimes infertility.

While a shocking number of women have endometriosis, it is an incredibly lonely, isolating illness. It is only recently that social media trends such as the 2018 campaign #1in10 have emerged and commercials on TV advertising new drugs and promoting awareness can be found. Although I've always preferred to remain private about my suffering—either physical or mental, I have found it therapeutic to write about my experience with endo. The very act of writing about my pain has helped me process it, come to terms with it, and, eventually, accept it as a part of me. Sharing my story has helped me feel less alone.

Cases of endometriosis are as different as the women who suffer from it. There are many complications of the illness ranging from degrees and types of pain, to depression and loss of quality of life. One thing we all have in common is that we suffer from a disease without a proven cure. I believe that since each case is different, so too is each effective treatment and path to healing. It is my hope that in sharing my experience with endometriosis and holistic medicine that people will find helpful solutions and take comfort in knowing that someone else understands what it feels like to suffer from a chronic disease. And perhaps, this book will set some on a curative path. Or, at least, let it be something solid to push either for or against.

1

THE BEGINNING

Every story has a beginning. This one has several. It could start with the first time I experienced pain and bleeding with intercourse. I was twenty-two, finishing college in Boston, and a casual encounter left me curled in post-coital agony. It could start a few years later when I began waking up in the middle of the night in severe left side pelvic and abdominal pain. I'd be up for an hour, sometimes more, desperately hugging a heating pad to my abdomen as I scrolled through Facebook looking for a distraction. It could also start in 2016 with a surgical procedure that yielded a diagnosis at thirty years old: I had endometriosis. But perhaps the most appropriate beginning for this story is at thirteen years old. After swimming in a friend's pool on a warm summer day, I found blood in my bathing suit: a first period.

Pre-pubescent, little girl features morphed into those of a young woman. Hips suddenly widened, curves appeared where before there was only scrawny, petite nothingness. A flat chest grew small, round breasts like white chrysanthemums sprouting from the earth. Fine, dark hair appeared in places that were previously smooth and doll-like. I began shaving my underarms and legs. Shirts and pants that used to hang loose on my small body filled out in flattering ways. And then, the final stroke of womanhood: menstruation.

Severe cramps and bloating came each month, unaffected by the Midol that my mother recommended. Mom instructed me to keep track of my cycle by writing the start and end dates of each period on the calendar. However, I quickly realized that my body rejected consistency. I complained to her and to my doctor about the discomfort and irregularity, and they responded that this was *just a part of being a woman.* The pain I endured each month was supposedly *normal.* In fact, through each of these first events, it was often dismissed. And, for seventeen years, I believed this lie: *a woman in pain is normal.*

In addition to the monthly discomfort, I was also very moody. Constantly irritable and desperately sad for no reason; I was a hormonal mess. As a product of a small parochial school, I learned about menstruation from a pamphlet and a one day, hour-long lesson that was reserved for the girls in the class. I found this booklet when I was sorting through old things during a move a few years ago. I perused the pages, written in diary form by a fictional girl named Kate. It covered the biology behind menstruation and included a list of the terms and definitions for female body parts and functions. The fictitious Kate speculated about when she might finally get her period and "average" girl issues such as liking boys, personal hygiene, and the moodiness that comes with such intense hormonal changes. Although I didn't expect this narrative to be particularly detailed, I was surprised by exactly how much was left out. There wasn't a single mention of cramps or of any physical symptoms that can occur with menstruation. Not a single reference. Kate's Diary conveyed the image of a painless period that might start out irregular at first but would eventually regulate, and the worst thing that would happen is weight gain and a little crankiness. Of course girls aren't prepared for what is, for some of us, the uncomfortable reality of a period. This sex education lesson was from the late 1990s, however, I suspect it hasn't evolved much since then.

I remember my mother signing a permission slip to attend the class. I remember I was eleven years old, and I remember the boys went to their own, separate session to learn about "boy things" from a male teacher. From such a young, impressionable age, I was taught that female health is not something to be shared with boys. It is uncomfortable, dirty, gross, embarrassing. But the lesson learned then went beyond shame. We learned that our bodies are all simple and the same, and because of this lack of complexity or difference, we only need one quick hour to educate us on the subject of puberty. Let's move through it as quickly and as cleanly as possible: these are the products you need; everyone's physical and mental symptoms will be the same; this is what it means to be a girl. There is no room for different experiences or dirty details. The devil, in this case, is certainly in the details. Give us the bare minimum so we aren't terrified when, one day, we find blood in our underwear. No, you aren't sick or dying. You might feel minor cramps, but they will go away. Deal with it. Okay, now off to math class.

I was reassured by my mother that the pain wouldn't last long or be too severe. Even the moodiness made sense, she said. But why do I feel like I'm standing on the edge of cliff and wanting to jump off? Why do I feel empty and so very sad? Why do I feel like a fist is clenched around my throat, and I can't breathe? Why do I cry when nobody is around? These are the questions I never thought to ask. I was alone and hurting. But I was only thirteen, hormones in overdrive, catapulted from girlhood to womanhood in the span of a year. And everyone left out those damn dirty details. So I must have been the freak show I believed I was, right?

And although endometriosis wasn't a part of my vocabulary yet, I can't help but wonder how I might have benefited from a more holistic approach to puberty. Would endo have remained nothing more than a stalker lurking around my organs, menacing, but ultimately not more than a threat? Would the sadness and anxiety have been managed better? Of course, these questions can never be answered. However, I can say that had I known this deluge of pain, confusion, and hormonal mutiny was coming, and had I been better equipped with proper tools and education, maybe it wouldn't have been so bad. Maybe my teen years would just be sparkling memories of drinking Starbucks in the parking lot with my friends, learning to drive my grandmother's Toyota Corolla, and silly inside jokes.

In the fall of 2004, I began college in Boston. A normal eighteen-year-old girl, I was in love with everything about this new life away from my hometown in Connecticut: the cosmopolitan crowds that lined the sidewalks of Commonwealth Avenue; the sound of the T as it rushed past vehicles and people, the loud creak of its doors opening and the electrical sparks spitting as it braked; rigorous classes taught in old Brownstones along the Charles River; and, of course, the sexual liberation afforded by birth control.

I recall walking along the Charles River in a hoodie and sweatpants, a coming-of-age cliché wearing innocence, wonder, and optimism like cheap accouterments purchased from the Claire's at the local mall. Some kids on roller blades passed by laughing. A band of pigeons crowded the walkway and got too close to my sneakers as I moved around them. Sitting on an empty bench overlooking the water, I pulled out my phone which wasn't yet a smartphone.

This was eighteen. The cool September air played with dark curly hair and ear buds blasted the soundtrack of early 2000s alternative rock: Coldplay, Foo Fighters, The White Stripes. I liked to drink rooibos lattes from a coffee shop on campus in those days, the days before it was all herbal teas and hot water. A book—likely *Baghavad Gita* or another ancient text from my freshman English class—laid open on my lap, the pages snapped in the breeze. These were the nuances of college life. But more than caffeinated beverages and intellectual reads, it was also a time for something equally adult: a first visit to Planned Parenthood.

Within a month of starting school, I had made an appointment at the local nonprofit organization. In my Catholic household, the name Planned Parenthood conjured images of sinful behavior and negative consequences. It meant premarital sex, sexually transmitted diseases, poverty, unspeakable sins. But as an eighteen-year-old college student, it meant affordable healthcare, condoms, birth control pills, and access to medical professionals who could offer the guidance I couldn't get from my mother's doctor back home. I walked there alone, through throngs of students and young professionals and protestors with signs extolling the virtue of human life. A flutter of wings filled my gut as I entered the building and was buzzed into the clinic.

I remember the crowded waiting room filled with women of all backgrounds and ages. A small TV played CNN and chairs with cracked brown leather seats scratched the backs of my legs. Before the physical examination, I was brought into a small room with a long, plastic folding table and harsh fluorescent lighting. The thirty-something, attractive nurse practitioner asked about my general health and any concerns I might have. I told her about my irregular periods and desire to go on birth control. Although I was still a virgin, I wanted to be ready for intercourse when the time and the right guy came along. This was the reason I wanted birth control and this is the reason the nurse gave me the samples and the prescription. No one thought twice about the fact that I had terrible cramps with menstruation or that my period would come every three weeks or sometimes five.

Perhaps it may seem like the silly, meaningless actions of a young woman, but the literal act of making an appointment at a place I imagined was forbidden by family, religion, and, even in some parts of the country, was freedom and womanhood. Taking a prescription for hormonal birth control pills would regulate my periods, allow me to become sexually active without fear of pregnancy, and even substantially reduce cramps and menstrual discomfort. At eighteen, this is what it meant to be *a normal woman*. For the first time since beginning my period at thirteen years old, I didn't experience nausea, cramps, bloating and fatigue each month. For the first time since I was thirteen years old, *I felt like a normal woman.*

I would manage for four years without any suspicion that endometriosis was lurking inside me. And when birth control pills no longer kept this chronic illness sedated, it would be years before I would know what was going on inside my body or how to fight back.

I did not know this then, but the agency afforded me as a young woman living in a Northeast city the first moment I had true control over my body. It wouldn't be the last, but I would lose—and eventually regain—that power. It would be taken by men, by disease, and by the very treatments intended to heal me. But during that first visit to Planned Parenthood I was truly liberated, and it was thrilling.

The next four years were virtually pain-free. I lost my virginity a year and a half after starting birth control. I fell in love, had my heart broken, engaged in casual sex. I encountered disappointment and hardship, made several enduring friendships, and in every way, had the opportunity to be a typical young woman. Birth control pills kept my monthly discomfort at bay and enabled me to lead a comfortable existence. That is, until one day, pain reentered my life like a thief—stealthy, unexpected, and determined to rob me of anything valuable.

2

BODY LIBERATED

The first time I experienced pelvic and abdominal pain was the night I cheated on Parker.

I met Parker during an interview for a hostess job at a local chain restaurant. He was a server there, ignoring his tables in favor of flirting with me. He found reasons to insert himself into my conversation with Neal, the corpulent manager with a scowl that should have been intimidating but was somehow softened by his off-color jokes. I was nineteen, in love with the idea of love, and struck by this man who wore a white seashell necklace and quoted *Family Guy* and *Shrek*. Undeniably Italian—olive skin, black buzzed hair, midnight sky eyes—he was a Hollywood handsome video gamer who loved comic books and curly-haired girls.

"You going to be the new hostess?" He asked, pen and pad still in hand from taking his table's order a few seconds earlier.

"Hopefully!" I replied, smiling as the restaurant soundtrack played Chicago's "Popsicle Toes."

"Giggity Giggity! Alllright!" The Family Guy reference caught me off guard, but I laughed.

From the moment I met him, I knew Parker was the one I wanted to give my virginity to. He was older than me by six years, and insecure despite his good looks. He was kind and funny, and loved Halloween and scary movies. I fell in love with him before we went on our first date.

We met in June and by September we were scribbling declarations of love in condensation in the rearview window of my Toyota Corolla. *I heart you.* We'd make out in his parked car, still wearing our work uniforms which smelled of fried food and sweat. I couldn't stand being apart from him for more than a couple days. We'd work together, hang out with friends at the diner and bar after work. I'd spend every night possible at his house, his parent's house, watching movies, eating Chinese takeout, and exchanging secrets and dreams. This was everything I believed love was: inside jokes, passionate kisses, and orgasms that literally made my toes curl. We were a Taylor Swift song playing on maximum volume. He taught me the pleasure my body could experience and the kind of pleasure I could give him. It was bliss and contentment—until it wasn't. Until I remembered he was six years older than me and talking about marriage and settling down. Until I cheated on him.

I lost my virginity to Parker on Valentine's Day in my college dorm room. I'd forgotten to make a dinner reservation so we ate a late meal at some dive bar in Brighton, a rather long walk from my dorm on West campus. The pub fare—meatloaf and mashed potatoes—was delicious but heavy. We walked it off as we made our way back to the tiny room on the twelfth floor. I remember when we kissed later that night, his mouth tasted like butter and garlic. When we removed our clothes, I remember I forgot to take off my socks. I felt silly still wearing them, but I was excited and nervous and figured he probably wasn't paying attention to my socks anyway. This was the moment that had been coming for the eight months we'd been together. And it was magical. For about five minutes.

But once we began having sex, we couldn't stop. We studied each other's bodies like tests we were desperate to ace or a foreign language we were learning to speak together. He taught me the kind of pleasure a woman can experience, and I was hooked. But I didn't just learn about pleasure—I learned about power. I was an average-looking, insecure girl with frizzy hair and too many imperfections to count. Sex with Parker was transformative; I became more confident in myself. Along with him, I learned the things my body could do and enjoy as well as the kind of things it could do to another body. This ability to give pleasure was intoxicating. For the first time in my life, I felt powerful. Through Parker, I learned that a woman's body can be revered; it's something sacred to be loved, adored, worshipped.

But ultimately, I was young. I made mistakes. And a relationship with that much heat will ultimately become a wildfire.

When I remember the night I cheated on Parker, I recall two things: the sudden, strange, crippling pain in my left side and a blood-stained pink Boston University t-shirt. These two distinct details persist even when the other specifics of the evening in May 2008 are more blurred lines on the edge of a photo than clear images.

Adam was five years older than me, tall and broad with wild, brown curls, and a reckless, scalding, sarcastic wit. He was intelligent, creative, and not my boyfriend. Our friendship began the summer before senior year when we worked together at the same restaurant where I met Parker who'd since taken a new job. We became friends from the first words we exchanged, likely a snarky comment from one or both of us.

Things between us changed when we traveled together after my college graduation. My friend Theresa and I had planned a European adventure—five countries, nine cities in four weeks. We purchased Eurail passes for the train, booked hostels, purchased suitcases and travel guides. Every detail was perfectly executed except for one: we wanted a third person, preferably a guy, to travel with us. We had no problem admitting that two twenty-two-year-old girls traveling alone could be targets for unsavory attention. This admission, we argued, did not make us less feminist, simply pragmatic. Adam was the ideal candidate for a third travel companion—imposing in stature, easygoing, and, mostly, available with a willingness to spend money on a four-week long European excursion.

Parker was not thrilled. We had been off-again-on-again for most of my college years, and one constant argument between us remained my friendship with Adam. He was jealous of our late night hang outs—drinking tea and hot chocolate in Roger's Park late into the night. He hated our easy banter and the long hours spent together at the restaurant. And he really hated the compliments he always gave me and the smiles that lingered long after the joke had expired. However, I was young and stubborn and despised being told what to do. Adam was just a friend, I insisted. And, at the time, I really meant it.

So I ignored Parker's protestations. When I went home for a long weekend during the planning phase of the trip, I invited Adam out to our usual spot for hot beverages. It was March then and cold at night so we kept the car running and the heat on. We parked by the black, stagnating pond where ducks would swim during daylight hours. A red brick municipal center complete with a basketball court was across the street. A large baseball field where youth sports teams played during baseball season was next to the pond. Street lamps lined the street and casted an orange-yellow glow like a row of artificial stars. These were the stars I wished upon as a coming-of-age twentysomething. I'd visit this spot often, with or without Adam, until the cops threatened us with a ticket for trespassing.

"Wanna run off to Europe with me?" I asked as I sipped hot black tea with milk from a Styrofoam cup.

Adam chuckled. "Yeah, sure."

"I'm serious. T and I are going day after graduation."

"Oh shit. For real?"

It didn't take much convincing. He committed to the trip before taking a first sip of his hot chocolate.

The night before we left for Logan airport and exactly two days after my graduation, Adam arrived at my red-brick, first-floor apartment in Brighton with his large suitcase. My own large suitcase –overstuffed and spilling clothes like a taco with too many fixings—occupied the center of my bedroom. He laughed at me, as all my friends did, for not understanding the art and nuance of packing light.

"So where are we drinking?" he asked, dropping his much smaller bag in the hallway.

What followed was an evening of tequila shots, draft beers, and warm white wine in a dimly lit basement bar in Allston. We were indefatigable then—the excitement of graduation, new adult jobs for some of us, impending adventure, and the energy of early twenties kept us up late socializing and imbibing. When we returned to the apartment after the bars closed and my girlfriends retired to their respective apartments, Adam and I sat together on the brown, velour couch from the 1980s that my parents had gifted me two years earlier.

I do not remember how words became kisses, but they did. One minute we were laughing about the fact that my roommates had to repack my suitcase and the next Adam's tongue was down my throat. His mouth tasted of beer and potato chips as the TV hummed in the background. My roommates weren't home and the place was dark, with the exception of the light from the television. I remember that I had changed into a light pink Boston University t-shirt with flannel pink plaid pajama pants. And when I retrace the lines of this evening, the night I cheated on my boyfriend with the friend he was jealous of, I fixate on this pink shirt.

I can still see spots of dried blood decorating the t-shirt in an odd, abstract pattern. I must have taken it off and thrown it on the couch as kissing became touching and touching became arousal and arousal became sex. We must have had sex on top of this shirt. While I don't recall its exact placement or the details of the sexual encounter, I do remember pain. And blood. The blood is a persistent detail of this night as powerful as the memory of the sudden overwhelming pain—like amplified cramps or something inside tearing, ripping apart like my insides were made of paper. Then the radiating, lingering pain twisting around inside for a few minutes only to disappear altogether as if it had never even happened, as if it was an apparition or phantom. The only evidence that it was real was the blood-stained pink t-shirt that I threw on the floor of my mostly empty bedroom.

I grabbed a pair of pajamas and curled up on the living room couch in a fetal position. Adam tried to be comforting, but I didn't want to cuddle, or, for that matter, be close to him. What was going on? Why was I experiencing such severe pain in my abdomen and pelvic area? This was not period pain, but what was it? I felt sick. While I didn't know much about female health, I did know that blood and pain during intercourse was not good. Something was wrong.

Part of me believed this pain was karmic. I had betrayed my boyfriend—the man who had loved me for three years. Guilt showed up the next morning like a hangover: overwhelming at first, but dissipating as the day went on. The initial nausea faded with a breakfast of bagels and the excitement of a pending European adventure. I tossed the pink T-shirt into a bag with the rest of my belongings to be washed or discarded later. I tossed the guilt aside too, to be dealt with when I returned from traveling for the next four weeks with the accessory to my moral crime.

Adam and I pretended as if nothing had happened for the majority of our trip. We were just a platonic trio making our way through museums and pubs and navigating the foreign roads and transit systems of Italy, Austria, Germany, Switzerland, and, finally, France. I didn't experience anymore pain or bleeding during this trip, and when Theresa left Adam and me in Paris to return home early—an attempt at cutting costs (we were, after all, broke twenty-something's)—we resumed where we had left off.

Parker was a continent away, and we were in Paris. Adam and I discovered a café by the hotel we were staying in in the Marmot district. The silver-haired, well-dressed bartender told us that "we are open until the sun comes up." The wine was cheap but delicious. We drank until we were hungry. There was a cart on the corner of the cobble-stoned street where a friendly Bangladeshi man in his late twenties sold bland pizza. After eating a slice or two, we watched as the sun began to come up over the still-energetic city. Adam and I went back to the small hotel room to get some sleep. Somehow, the room we booked only had a single bed with limited floor space. Adam was over six feet tall, and, although he offered to sleep on the floor, it would be nearly impossible for him to get any rest in such a cramped space. I gave him permission to share the bed with me. Thoughts of Parker were muted by too much wine and distance. This was Paris, the city of love. I was twenty-two, a budding writer, a romantic, a young woman looking for adventure stories I could scribe in my newly purchased journal. Adam was a man I connected with emotionally—I could tell him anything and everything; Parker was pressuring me to commit in ways I couldn't.

I tossed and turned. Adam tossed and turned beside me. Dawn slipped into the room through the open window. I turned away from the pinkish gold light, from his body breathing hard under the thin white sheet. I faced the wall. I focused on slowing my breath

13

which sounded loud in the quiet room. The only other sound was his breathing—just as loud, just as fast.

"You awake?" He asked finally, after what seemed like hours.

"Yes." I rolled over to face him.

Before either of us said anything else, he kissed me.

Drunk sex became a ritual every night we shared a bed in Paris. Five nights of drinking wine until sunrise followed by amorous activities in the tiny hotel room turned my old friend into a new lover. It surprised me how natural making love to Adam was. Our bodies seemed to fit together like two halves of a friendship locket. But the pain inside me was lurking, waiting while I hurt the man I loved with another man I also might have loved. And endometriosis was waiting to exact its revenge.

When I came back from Europe, I didn't want to have sex with Parker. I had spent a week sleeping with my best friend, and it continued when we were back home. We attempted to recreate Paris in late-night wine binges at his condo while we watched episodes of an HBO show called Rome. Two, three glasses of cheap chardonnay in and we'd find ourselves laughing at Lucius and Titus—the main characters of the historical drama. I don't know if the show about Ancient Rome was actually funny or not. We never made it through a full episode before he'd touch my leg or brush his hand against my cheek. Our faces and bodies inevitably ended up pressed against each other as the sound of battles and unfolding political intrigue played out on the screen.

But my own battle and tale of intrigue was playing out in the real world. Although I was sleeping with Adam, I was also starting to experience pain on occasion which was the excuse I used to avoid intercourse with Parker. I told him I felt pain and nausea; he would pout and try talking me into sex, but, ultimately, he gave up.

I eventually ended both relationships. Adam and I continued to be friends although we weathered a few rough months after he accused me of using him to make myself feel better about the deteriorating relationship with Parker. Parker, on the other hand, did not take the breakup well. He continued to pursue me which only drove me further away. But Parker would not completely exit my life for a couple more years; he was like a stress cigarette when I'd been smoke-free for months. I always picked him up again, craving, needing that hit of nicotine.

3

BODY IN DISTRESS

Something is wrong. I told the doctor at my next gynecological visit about my symptoms which had become more frequent. Explosions of severe, sharp jabs on my left side, like blades piercing, cutting slowly away at my organs interrupted my days and nights. She insisted that it was probably an untreated STD. I was a twenty-three-year-old sexually active female so, naturally, this must be the culprit. The doctor did raise the possibility of ovarian cysts, but, she explained, they would have ruptured already or would rupture on their own, and they were much less likely.

I was reassured by this older, female doctor. She was, after all, an expert with years of experience in the medical field. Her maternal characteristics—soft face, a fan of lines around her eyes that fluttered when she smiled, and her use of terms of endearment like "sweetie"—exuded wisdom and comfort. If this kind woman thought everything was fine, then it must be fine. Even though the STD tests came back clear and the pain during sex and occasional bleeding continued, I subscribed to her casual tone and lack of general worry. After all, *a woman in pain is normal,* isn't it?

This was the state my body was in when it suffered another attack; but this one was personal and from an external enemy. It was a busy Friday night shift during the holidays. The restaurant was located in a mall and since holiday shopping had commenced, hungry, tired people packed the place. I can't remember what I needed in dry storage, but I had gone into the room off the kitchen filled with boxes of napkins, extra bottles of ketchup, salt and pepper, and a sundry of other items. Two men—co-workers, people I had liked, joked around with in between trips to my tables—followed me into the room, closed the door behind them, and shut off the light.

As they took turns forcing their hands in my shirt, down my pants, and covering my mouth, I screamed for someone, anyone to help. But, like so many often do, my voice got lost; it was just another sound in a cacophony of kitchen noises: the sizzling of pans, cooks laughing, servers yelling for food, utensils clinking against plates, and me, my small, muffled voice crying out from a darkened room.

I didn't realize it then, but like many victims of sexual assault, my attitude towards sex and my body changed afterwards. Pain and denial made me cruel; I became a succubus. I sought out men to be broken with and to break, other puzzle pieces whose edges I could try to fit into my own. But I didn't view them as equals; they were cardboard-cut-out boys I could fold, bend, and shred at my leisure. Toys for entertainment.

This stage—reckless, casual, desperate, power-hungry sex—was a chapter of my life filled with lines I don't like to reread, ones I'd prefer to skim over or ignore all together. However, these lines, these moments are vital to my story's plotline. My body became a tool for experiencing pleasure—a pleasure I needed and yearned for and pursued with an almost fanatical persistence. This need for attention and love was unhealthy, but I craved it perhaps because during this time, I'm not sure I loved myself.

I was heartbroken, vulnerable, angry, desperate, promiscuous. Although intercourse became painful at times and orgasms were especially excruciating, I did my best to ignore it and continue with my sexual escapades. And besides, the pain was not consistent or ubiquitous yet; it popped into my life on occasion like a long-distance, offensive relative —unexpected, unwelcome, and very unpleasant. But, at this point, it never remained for more than a few days at a time, and I could go months without so much as a flare-up.

During this time, I experimented with a second means of coping with trauma. I would like to say that I started taking Oxycodone to manage my physical pain, but that would be a lie. I dabbled in pain killers as a means of a different kind of pain management before endo-metriosis took center stage in my life. I was aching for more—more travel, more professional satisfaction, more—better—love. When Parker and I broke up again, I was heartbroken. I had also just been sexually assaulted at work. These two unrelated events happened within the same month, and I wasn't able to cope with either of them in a healthy manner. The bottle of Oxycodone pills in the back of a drawer in my sister's room, leftover from her wisdom teeth extraction, tucked beneath summer tops she didn't need for autumn in Massachusetts, summoned me from a restless sleep. Like a sailor following the songs of the Sirens, I made my way to her bedroom, to the rocky coast I could wreck myself on. The small orange bottle with its childproof white cap and insides filled with enchanting white pills felt big in my cold, clammy hands. What music would you play for me, little Siren pills? What mythological experience can you give me? Can you save me from the abyss inside my head? The sea storm raging inside my heart?

When I was sexually assaulted at twenty-three, I swallowed it and the secret made the hole inside me deeper and darker. I acted out. I cheated on the man I loved with men I didn't. We broke up and got back together and he called twenty-three times and we fought and I yelled and he cried and we fell into the bottom of each other's souls and got lost. When we broke up the last time, the pain inside was too much. I took pills and liked them. I realized I could kill myself without actually dying. Oxycodone. I became blissfully numb. My body didn't hurt; my mind didn't hurt; my soul didn't hurt. I'd been gutted by two men who put their hands in my shirt and down my pants in a storage room at work. I'd been gutted by a breakup. First assault or first love—each is a syndrome, a curse. I was inconsolable. He said he loved someone else. I took the bottle of Oxycodone pills and popped a few one night before bed. I couldn't feel anything at all. No sadness. No broken heart. No love.

And then I was no longer a girl in pain. Until I was. When the drugs and drinks and sex wore off, I was broken and jagged again—a piece of glass for boys to cut themselves on. I liked hurting them; it felt good to inflict pain on others. I wouldn't be alone in my suffering then. I was a girl in pain, but I'd make others hurt too. I spun a gray cocoon around myself and refused to emerge. The butterfly I could become shriveled up and died.

The first night I took one pill. I popped it into my mouth, swallowed it without water, and returned to my bed to let its effects wash over me. It didn't take long before I could feel the nothingness. My external body was immune to any kind of feeling but so too, was my internal self. Heartache and anxiety dissipated. I was numb but also I was left with a calm sensation unlike anything I'd ever experienced. This was bliss. This was peace. This was contentment.

I repeated this act the next night and the next until it became a bedtime ritual. Say goodnight to my mother, brush my teeth, get into pajamas, sneak into my little sister's room, take a pill or two, return to bed, and drift off to a world without pain. My Narnia, my Elysium, my Garden of Eden.

After some weeks of taking pills, I began to lose weight. I couldn't keep food down. My stomach often hurt, and I didn't feel hungry. When I did eat, it was only small amounts, and I typically had to excuse myself to the bathroom before the meal was over so that I could vomit. I began to look pale and tired and, as one coworker commented, like I had just been released from a concentration camp. This should have been alarming. This should have scared me into stopping, but, unfortunately, I was hooked on the feeling of not feeling. I counted the minutes until I could go home and get high.

When my supply ran out after a few weeks, I tried to find more. I worked in a restaurant, and many of my co-workers were big partiers. If they didn't do Oxy themselves, they certainly knew people who did. I didn't realize it at the time, but these people were good friends. They suspected I was abusing pain killers, and they made it impossible for me to purchase. Until Miles began working as a server.

Miles and I connected from the moment he began working with me. He was funny and easy to talk to and mostly, he loved snorting Oxy. He was also a dealer. When he learned of my quest, he was only too happy to help. He offered me a new sufficient supply for fifty dollars. I turned over my money to this guy I only knew for a week without so much as a second thought.

But then Miles disappeared with the money. I heard he'd been arrested in Vermont, but I could never really be sure what happened to him. All I know for certain is Miles became the best cautionary tale I never asked for. I had been robbed of fifty dollars and withdrawal had already begun. I deleted him from my phone, and embraced the cold sweats and waves of vomiting.

Because I had gone down the medication path already and it was the rain-slicked road I crashed on, when endometriosis pain seized my organs, I couldn't take real pain killers. When I would lie awake in the middle of the night with crippling pelvic and abdominal pain and corresponding painsomnia, the only option available to me was Tylenol or Aleve—which didn't even take the edge off. The ineffectiveness of over-the-counter drugs coupled with the fear of taking more potent pain killers and liking them seemed to leave me with no options for pain management.

One Saturday during a busy lunch shift, I doubled over in sudden and severe abdominal and pelvic pain. It was overwhelming. I suffered through the shift, clutching my left-side and squatting on the kitchen floor to catch my breath. I remember trying to bring a tray of food to a table of customers when the pain, which had been consistent throughout the day, suddenly spiked. If it had been playing all day at a soft, throbbing tempo, this was punched up to maximum volume. The pain in my left side was deafening; I couldn't focus or hear or process the other servers laughing around me, the cooks yelling to each other in Spanish, or the loud rush of patrons just beyond the front server station. I sat on the floor, holding and pressing my stomach and left side as if I could simply smother it. When it didn't go away after a half hour or so, I asked to be cut early so I could go to the hospital.

The emergency room waiting area was filled with people. A young Hispanic woman with a coughing toddler, a fifty-something man with shaking hands and a reddish face, and a young boy, probably around seven or eight, in a soccer uniform cradling his arm with watery eyes, his impatient and irritable parents chiding the woman at the front desk for making them wait. Then there was me. I had changed from my uniform—black pants and blue collard shirt—into yoga pants and a long-sleeved tee.

I waited and waited and waited. Then I was called into a room to be assessed by a nurse who took my vitals and asked about my sexual history. She explained that I was likely experiencing complications of an STD. This was not the first time a medical professional, always a woman, assumed that my pelvic and abdominal discomfort was the result of the fact that I was sexually active. If a woman is sexually active, she must be a slut. If she's a slut and in pain, she must have a sexually transmitted disease. This is the attitude a twentysomething woman is faced with today. This is often the judgment she endures not from her peers or parents, but from the people who are supposed to help her feel better.

After the initial intake, I was sent to another room to wait some more. Another hour or two passed and a frazzled, middle-aged doctor rushed into see me. She spent a few minutes basically asking the same questions the nurse had several hours earlier, echoed her conclusion, but decided that it didn't hurt to have an intravaginal ultrasound to rule out any potential serious problems. She seemed to proscribe this test as an afterthought, as if my pain couldn't possibly be the result of an actual medical issue. This doubt, this dismissal by a doctor in a hospital seemed to amplify the pain or at least the emotional anguish. I wiped tears away from my eyes, slumped forward in the cold, leather chair in this room with curtains for walls and waited once again.

Blistering pain, searing, crippling—I searched my repertoire of words, seeking just the right one. But it didn't exist. This pain transcended language. It was ineffable. I thought that perhaps my inability to effectively articulate this pain was the reason I was brushed off by the doctor, discharged, and sent home with nothing more than a handout about ovarian cysts that was printed by a printer running out of ink, the words black and blurred as I tried to read them from tearing eyes which certainly didn't help. The intravaginal ultrasound revealed fluid—remnants of an ovarian cyst that had already ruptured.

"The pain should be over now. Go home and take Aleve. You'll be fine." The doctor told me as she handed me discharge papers.

I felt like nothing more than a used tissue tossed into a trash can— useless, forgettable, inconsequential. This is what my pain was to her. This is what I was to her. A silly, useless, forgettable girl whose pain should be gone and if it wasn't then obviously an over-the-counter drug should fix it. It hadn't occurred to her that I'd already tried over-the-counter pain killers and they had failed, which is why I was in the emergency room in the first place. But, then, I suppose it hadn't occurred to her, quite simply, because she didn't care. I didn't matter. My pain didn't matter.

In all likelihood, she probably wasn't as heartless or indifferent as my memory has rendered her. She was likely busy, tired, overworked, and perhaps even unaware of what other possible conditions could be ailing me. Endometriosis wasn't a word that ever touched the lips of any doctor I'd encountered then, and, even now, it trips out of their mouths, clumsy, like they aren't sure it's anything more than voodoo witchcraft concocted by mystics or artists or feminists, but it exists, they're pretty sure, and they tolerate it.

But it was 2009 then. It had been a full year since my first painful episode. And this was the ordeal I endured for the next six years as the pain escalated. In 2015, I was twenty-nine and coming apart like a spider web in the wind. I was fragile and powerless against the apathy I encountered with each doctor I visited. Innumerable waiting rooms—all marked by the same stiff chairs and fluorescent lights and stacks of old magazines on end tables—filled the months. A dizzying montage of doctors and exams and misdiagnoses followed. A middle-aged balding gastroenterologist who dismissed me from the moment he entered the exam room; the prettier, also middle aged, female gastroenterologist who was certain I had irritable bowel syndrome or definitely something digestive and who ordered a colonoscopy and endoscopy and seemed truly perplexed when everything came back normal; the affable Indian gynecologist who was convinced it must be muscular and thought I should see a surgeon, whom I ignored completely; the curt, curly-haired nurse practitioner who thought it could be something serious like cancer and thought I should get blood work. The sweet, chatty gynecologist who finally suggested

24

it could be endometriosis who proscribed a different birth control pill that could manage the pain but, who, when these pills caused my hair to fall out in clumps and didn't help with the pain at all, ignored my calls like a bitter ex-lover; and who, finally, had a nurse call me back and instruct me to continue taking these pills. There were other doctors and emergency room visits and serious tests all without results or progress. There was even WebMD whom I turned to in utter desperation only to learn that the website was certain I had a rare cancer based on the symptoms I'd entered into the search, and I was likely going to die.

January 2016, one month before my thirtieth birthday, I had been dealing with near constant, crippling pain. One blustery morning, I woke up in such agony that I had to cancel classes for the day. I was an adjunct professor teaching writing at several universities in Connecticut. Most days, I taught through the pain. I'd lock myself in the bathroom on campus in between classes to catch my breath until the episode became manageable. This day was different. The pelvic and abdominal pain was unbearable. Nothing helped, and I had reached a breaking point. I sobbed in the car as I drove myself to the emergency room. At this time, I still had no answers as to what was causing my pain. On this particular afternoon, I was heading to the hospital equally desperate for pain relief and answers. What I got was this: after waiting for hours, after yet another intravaginal ultrasound which came back clean, the doctor sent me home with instructions to take Aleve and follow up with my gynecologist. *Take Aleve.* I waited for hours only to be told to do what I had already done. Medication didn't even take the edge off of the pain. I had already lost count of the number of doctors I'd seen. It is impossible to convey the frustration, anger, desperate sadness that one experiences in this moment. There are no words appropriate or strong enough to convey the exact feelings that correlate with being dismissed with the medical equivalent of a pat on the head. I was on a carousel of nightmarish horses going around and around and around and around. And I wanted off.

Finally, after almost a year of continuous pain and zero progress with doctors, I saw a gynecologist who was confident I had endometriosis and she was ready to take a serious step which would, theoretically, confirm diagnosis and relieve the pain: she wanted to perform a laparoscopy.

This serious, but pleasant woman with a round face and blue eyes that reminded me of summer skies and youth and days before pain explained the procedure in the small, white exam room. It was the first visit with this gynecologist, and I appreciated her let's-get-down-to-it attitude; she was almost arrogant as she told me the procedure was minimally-invasive, primarily diagnostic, but if she saw evidence of endometriosis, which she was sure she would, she'd simply remove it, and all would be well. This sounded like the fairy-tale ending I had spent the past year searching for—girl meets doctor, girl gets diagnosis, doctor saves girl from a life of pain, girl lives happily ever after.

I should have known happy endings are only for bedtime stories and Disney princesses.

4

BODY IN PAIN

My body in pain was a stranger I'd never met. A bad one-night stand who refused to leave. At first, it was a smattering of days that stabbed, hurt, inconvenienced and then dissipated. And then they became consistent and consistently bad; a new routine I never wanted. The pain spilled over the minutes and hours of my days like a blot of dark ink, eventually blocking out the images of anything else. Pain so hot it turned my skin ice cold.

I can count the number of times I missed work from endometriosis on one hand, but that's not to say that I felt well enough to work. Accepting that my body was rebelling against me, and that, maybe, I wasn't the same woman I had always been, was challenging. I didn't know how to navigate the day while the disease wreaked havoc on my organs. I had sex even though it was often uncomfortable, even painful. I went out with my friends, drank wine on girls' nights, cleaned the house, and continued writing at my favorite coffee shops. Most of the time, I remained amiable and focused. In the beginning, the relationship I had with my body was unchanged: I lived as if nothing about me was different even though nothing was the same.

For a long time, I resisted identifying myself as a woman in chronic pain. I would not let this illness become my Svengali, pulling my strings as if it could own me.

Some days trying to stay sane was like running drunk with a stack of china. There were mornings I woke with dark clouds beneath my eyes; this was when the pain pinched me awake and shook me till sleep was impossible. Painsomnia. Insomnia plus pain equals waking nightmare. These were the nights I spent watching TV shows I'd seen a dozen times in the hope that they'd lull me back to sleep. These were the nights I laid on the bathroom floor with my blue heating pad waiting for my organs to stop shattering. These were the nights I spent scrolling through social media, looking for interesting articles or funny memes to make me laugh when laughter was something that seemed like a relic of an ancient past, an artifact buried under miles of sleep.

I became adept at playing pretend. I stole moments of my day and hid inside them: curling into the fetal position on the floor of my office with the lights out so that no one would suspect I was there and dare to knock; squatting in the bathroom stall of the ladies' room on campus with my fist in my mouth, biting down so I didn't scream in pain; brushing away the tears of the most recent episode while forcing a bright smile as I walked into my classroom to teach freshman composition. During these painful moments, I focused on happier times. I remembered being a child playing dolls with my two younger sisters; my dad cooking pancakes on Sunday mornings before church; the first time I had a short story published. I swallowed these memories like pain killers and sometimes they even gave me enough of a buzz to get through the agony.

I tried to treat the pain the way the doctors suggested. I took over-the-counter painkillers like Aleve. They did nothing. I used a heating pad which didn't really help but made me feel somewhat relaxed until the direct application of heat printed a bright red splotch on my belly like a slap. I took birth control pills. Some pills made my hair fall out in clumps leaving bald spots and clogging the shower drain. Other pills made me emotional, volatile, like I was a live grenade and a simple breath on my neck would cause me to detonate.

What is it like to be a working body in pain? It is like having a secret, a bad habit, you don't want anyone to know about. It's the cigarette breath you conceal with mint gum. But there is no discernable scent of endometriosis pain and the only noticeable trace of it would likely be the occasional grimace I can't conceal or the dried tears I didn't quite brush away. I kept my pain to myself; I never felt like it was something that belonged in my work place, not because my co-workers and superiors wouldn't be understanding or supportive, but simply because chronic pain had already invaded the other areas of my life. It was a part of my personal space, a visible plateau in my emotional landscape. It often dominated my sex life—dictating when I could and couldn't make love. It controlled my sleep—preventing me from getting a restful night whenever it flared. I would not allow it to take my work from me too. I loved teaching college students. I loved conversing with my colleagues in the hallway between classes. I loved the act of writing and revising, creating artful sentences, dabbing at them until they were beautiful pages. Endometriosis would not take this from me; I wouldn't let it.

This reluctance on my part meant that I almost never missed a day of work. I almost never cancelled class. If a wave of pain came on during a lesson, I breathed through it, concentrated on the ideas I was sharing with my students. I'd also usually sit in a chair in the front of my classroom slightly bent forward, elbows propped on a table in front of me. To the students, this was nothing significant; to me, it was the most comfortable position I could get myself into without betraying the pain raging inside my body.

Endometriosis did not just impact my work day, it also sometimes affected my commute. More times than I can count, I'd experience a scene like this: I am driving to work, and I really have to pee. I had peed before I left the house—twice—but my frequent consumption of tea along with the natural frequency of urination that correlates to this disease—has resulted in a full bladder before I've reached campus. This is bad. Why? Because a full bladder on a pain day equals really bad flare. I can feel the cramping, searing sensation begin when I am about five minutes away from my destination. The pain amps up and climaxes as I am still driving, pulling into the parking lot. I manage a smile and wave to the parking lot attendant even though I feel like my bladder is a balloon filled with too much helium and it's about to pop. The pain tightens around it, a fist squeezing this organ that's already about to burst. Thankfully, the pain subsides somewhat as I park and exit my vehicle. I rush to the bathroom, relieve myself, and savor the emptiness, the pain powering down. Relief.

A body in pain shouldn't be normal, but sometimes it is. I did not know how to accept this truth and it made me depressed but also angry. It made me so angry that I fought. I refused to give in to the pain and the difficulty and the constant struggle of getting through a day without breaking into pieces like the porcelain doll I felt I'd become. I would find answers and then solutions. There had to be answers and solutions. This was the 21st century. There had to be answers. There had to be solutions.

5

CHRONIC: A LOVE STORY

There is a statue of Juliet near The Old Town Hall between Marien-platz and the Viktualienmarkt in Munich, Germany. The bronze statue of Shakespeare's heroine was a gift from the city of Verona in the early 1970s. Local lore instructs its visitors to leave her flowers so that they might have luck in finding true love. I heard this story on a walking tour of Munich when I spent a few days there in 2008. And as a young woman of twenty-two, a recent college graduate filled with romantic ideals and a slowly-breaking heart, this bit of local legend appealed to me.

On my last day in the German city, I left my friends behind in the hostel so that I could pay homage to the statue. I remember buying a single pink rose from a vendor with a stand set up in the bustling central square. Surrounding purveyors offered samples of cheeses, mustards, and jams. The salty scent of freshly baked pretzels mixed with a sweet floral aroma in the damp air. The day was gray, teetering on the edge of cold, and a soft rain began to fall as I approached her. Juliet was covered in brightly-colored bouquets, some lay at her base, others filled the crook of her arm. How many sad and longing would-be lovers had made this pilgrimage before me, I wondered, placing my flower beside the bronze hem of her dress. I looked into her empty eyes and asked her to send me my soul mate. The rain picked up before I left, running cold down the back of my neck, trailing along my skin like fingertips.

Exactly one year and seven months later, I walked into an Irish Pub in my Connecticut hometown. I was not supposed to be at this bar; I'd made plans with a couple friends to have a quiet evening of cocktails elsewhere but a last minute addition of several people and some cajoling from my aspiring attorney friend, and I somehow ended up at a rowdy bar with loud live music and too many people for my mood. I was tired from waitressing a busy day shift, and I was still recovering from the most recent breakup with my on-again, off-again boyfriend. I did not feel friendly or flirty; I did not want to dance or drink too much. And I certainly did not plan to meet my future husband.

Waiting to order a Vodka cranberry while the bartender chatted with two pretty brunettes, I plopped my large white purse down on the oak colored bar. An attractive, dark-haired man with a goatee looked over at me and said, "Way to bring your duffle bag to the bar."

"It's actually a mini-duffle bag, thank you very much." I smiled at my witty retort.

He laughed.

I don't recall the dialogue that came next, but I do remember how easy it was to talk to this stranger, how familiar he felt although we'd never met. I remember that I told him I had aspirations of becoming a writer, and he asked if I had written anything.

"Yes, but nothing has been published."

"Well, that doesn't matter. You write so you're a writer."

Such simple, straightforward logic. So practical. Like the way he rolled up the sleeves of his collared shirt to reveal strong arms covered in dark hair. Or his oil-stained finger nails. Or his hazel eyes, a shade of brown with flecks of green, the color of the earth, the trees, the forest I could get lost in. He was not complicated like poetry or bad-habit ex boyfriends; This man was whiskey, straight up.

It was January then, cold in Connecticut, but for the week after I met Greg I was warm anytime I thought about him. He called the next day at the end of my lunch shift. I was still in uniform, apron heavy with wads of dollar bills, loose change, order pad, and several pens. In the middle of rolling silverware for the nightshift, my cell phone vibrated indicating a new voicemail. My heart rate accelerated, and I had to remember to breathe.

I liked Greg, that much was clear. But I was hesitant. I was on the cusp of twenty-four, waiting to hear back from graduate programs and figuring out next steps. It was 2010, and I was nearing two years since I'd graduated from college. I couldn't seem to gain any traction professionally, however, I was motivated to sift some direction from the scraps of this post-collegiate life. There were options to consider: Continue waitressing? Apply for entry-level jobs in publishing or journalism? Move to New York City? Entering a new relationship didn't make the list, and I had closed the chapter on casual hookups.

Ultimately, the only reason I agreed to a first date with Greg was because of a dream. My deceased grandmother visited me in my dreams on occasion, especially before I had to make a major life decision. Going on a date with some guy I met at an Irish pub certainly didn't seem to qualify as a major life event, however, Grandma Mary appeared to me nonetheless one night a few days after our first phone chat. I don't recall the specifics of the dream, but, now, even more than a decade later, I can clearly remember that she warned me, in uncharacteristically ominous tone: If you don't go on a date with Greg, you will regret it for the rest of your life. Well, shit. That seemed a little melodramatic, but I was not about to piss off my nocturnal ghost grandma. I texted him the next morning: *I'm free Friday night.*

He responded: *I'll pick you up at 7:30.*

If I hadn't gone out with Greg, if I'd blown him off in favor of the bad habit ex-boyfriend or the pipe dream city apartment—my grandmother was right—I would have regretted it for the rest of my life. Because Juliet had sent me my soul mate. And while Greg may not believe in signs, luck, fate, phantoms, or magic statues, I believe I married the man of my dreams because of a bronze German sculpture and my dead grandmother.

Greg would say it was because his joke about my purse was hilarious.

In the early years of dating, we could enjoy passionate intercourse without more than just a sporadic burst of pain. However, after a few years, the pain become a third-party in our relationship, a ménage a trois no one wanted. It disrupted our sex life to the point where I stopped enjoying sex. Even when we could make love without interruption, an intense flare-up would inevitably follow. I could expect to spend any intimate post-coital moments in tears with a heating pad to my belly instead of resting in Greg's arms. To his credit, he was understanding and supportive. He'd offer at late hours to run to the CVS to get medicine or relocate to the couch so I could spread out more comfortably in bed. His hazel eyes revealed more than concern in those moments; they had distinct notes of guilt. I knew he couldn't help but feel as though he had caused my pain. I can't imagine what it must feel like to watch your partner curl up in agony after making love with you—that is an entirely different brand of hurt.

By 2015, the pain evolved into a permanent shadow, and a restful night's sleep became an impossible goal. Nearly every night I woke at least once or twice from a deep sleep because the pain radiating inside me exploded like a firecracker, and startled me out of the deepest of sleep. I'd grab the heating pad I started leaving by my bedside—it had become a fixture, part of the nightstand's décor—and walk to the living room so as not to wake Greg. I'd lay on the couch, throw a blanket over me, and take out my phone to scroll through Facebook. *Who else is awake at 3:00 a.m.*, I wondered. *Maybe I could find an interesting article to pass the time? I could watch another episode of Criminal Minds on Netflix.* When the morning finally came, I felt as though I hadn't slept at all. It always seemed that when the pain lessened or disappeared long enough for me to fall back to sleep, it was invariably time to wake up and start the day. I was exhausted all the time.

When I was just a girl dreaming of love and wishing for it on shooting stars and birthday cakes, I imagined grand romantic gestures like a dozen roses for no reason and poetic avowals in the middle of a rainstorm. But real life looks different from the romanticized notions of little girls still growing up. In place of fancy jewelry or dinner at a nice restaurant, it is the thoughtful things that make me fall in love with Greg more every day. It is the TENS machine he brought home from work because he heard it could help with endometriosis pain. It's the way he gets out of bed in the middle of the night when I'm having an episode to find my heating pad or the way he offers to brew me a cup of tea even though he's never made a cup of tea in his life. It's the way he holds me tightly when I'm in pain and we can't do anything else.

And I especially appreciate the way he makes me laugh.

Greg proposed on a Tuesday night during an episode of NCIS. I wasn't entirely sure he had asked me to marry him, in fact, as there was no clear question, more of a vague statement about the future and marriage.

"Wait, was that a proposal? Do you want to get married?" I asked as I turned away from the characters examining a crime scene, dead body sprawled across the screen.

"Sure, why not?" Every girl's dream proposal.

We eloped the next month in Punta Cana.

It is 2022 now. We've been married for five years, together for twelve. Endometriosis doesn't feel like an unwanted guest in our relationship anymore. It is still there, but it's no longer omnipresent. It will always be an extra in our lives, lingering in the wings. An afterthought. A shadow inhabiting the fringes of our days, no longer casting a cloud over them.

Now, he walks behind me and grabs my butt as I'm brushing my teeth before bed. I laugh because I'm embarrassed at the reflection in the mirror. Messy bun—dark curls piled high, a halo of frizz not quite contained by the hair tie, makeup free complexion imperfect—a large pimple center of my chin—oversized t-shirt that hides the suggestion of curves. I am the opposite of sexy. I am end-of-the-day, working mom of a toddler, mid-endo flare attractive; that is to say, I've looked better.

He grabs my butt again, making his amorous intentions clear.

Laughing again, I spit a glob of toothpaste into the sink and say, "Honey, I'm so gross right now."

"You're beautiful." He says as he moves his hands around my waist. "And Bertha is in rare form tonight," He adds, referring to the massive zit on my face.

"I'm having a bad pain day." I lean into his embrace, appreciative of the attention even if I'm not feeling remotely interested in sexual activity.

"So if that part's broken, does that mean we can try the other hole?" His eyes meet mine in the mirror and smile. We both laugh.

"Nice try."

"So that's a yes?" He smirks, knowing the answer is no but not passing up an opportunity to joke about butt stuff. "It could help, you know. It would qualify as holistic, right?"

We laugh again. I worry we might wake our daughter who is asleep in the next room.

"Butt sex as the new endo treatment?"

"I bet it would be really popular with husbands!"

"I'm sure it would."

"Although FDA approval might be hard to get."

"Most likely."

We stand in the bathroom and laugh until the dog wakes up and glares at us from his bed.

6

THE EPIPHANY

I remember lying in bed in Norwalk Hospital after surgery. The sheets were stiff and cold, and I was lightheaded and nauseous. Images of people—my parents, nurses—floated around me like faded memories. The anesthesia was wearing off, and I was groggy, but the smile on the doctor's face was vivid as she told me, "We got it; we got all of it." Although moments later I'd be vomiting and trying not to pass out in the tiny private bathroom off of my room, I felt something familiar twisting in my chest: hope. *My endometriosis was gone. My pain would be gone. I would no longer be a woman in pain.*

For almost eight years I'd suffered. Some days it felt like hot coals sat inside my abdomen. The heat—red hot pain heat—melted everything inside and I could feel every burn, every flame, every scar as it was forming. The coals rolled around inside me often finding their way to my backside, searing my rectum so that it felt as though the organ itself was tearing like wrapping paper. My cheeks would burn too. I'd sweat and breathing became forced. Tears would well in my eyes. The pain was everything, all of me, all-consuming, all-powerful. It was as if my body was governed by a deranged and sadistic god. This surgery was my revolt, my revolution against this cruel dictator. I felt like a mighty warrior, albeit one who was pale, shaking and vomiting in the bathroom of a hospital, adorned in thick, slip-resistant hospital socks and a flimsy gown that wouldn't stay tied.

The doctor discharged me after a few hours. Still nauseous, abdomen sore from the fresh incisions on each side and inside my belly button, I pulled my yoga pants on and a sweatshirt. I remember nodding off to sleep in the back seat of my mother's Toyota as she drove me to her place. It was a dreamless, heavy sleep—the kind I rarely seemed to get anymore. The months leading up to the laparoscopy were filled with long nights spent awake, in pain, watching Netflix or scrolling through social media on my phone while Greg slept soundly in the next room. I'd spend an hour, sometimes less, laying on the couch in the living room, heating pad plugged in and hot on my bare stomach. I always turned the heat on so high that it would turn my belly red, perhaps because a part of me felt as if I could drive the pain away with excessive heat. Unfortunately, all it ever did was burn my skin.

Recovering from the excision surgery and ablation was not easy. During the procedure, air is pumped into your body. Afterwards, that gas causes extreme pain in your shoulders. I had to force myself to walk around the house to break up the gas bubbles, a feat which was unpleasant as my incisions were sore, and I was still experiencing abdominal and pelvic pain. Movement, though necessary, was exhausting and uncomfortable.

A week post-op, I was lying in bed, in the dark, attempting to distract myself from the pain with the TV.

"The pain is just as bad as before," I sobbed into the phone. The voice of the physician seemed to reveal confusion, frustration, and skepticism. She performed the procedure and was confident everything was removed. I imagined a debate was raging in her head: was I lying? Did I just want pain meds? She reluctantly prescribed pain killers, but stopped short of giving me narcotics. She made it apparent in her severe tone that she didn't believe pain medication was necessary, and she didn't like the idea of giving them to me one bit.

I had no interest in drugs. I was single-minded in what I wanted: recovery. Pain-free existence without drugs of any kind. I wanted to be normal. I wanted my life back. I didn't want to deal with doctors anymore—the good ones or the bad. I wanted to be done with it all. And she had told me it was over, I was healed. *She got all of it,* she had boasted post-op. The very real pain tearing up my insides suggested otherwise.

I wasn't supposed to drive for a week and I couldn't lift anything heavy which included my school bag, however, I was not one for missing work. I had already canceled two days of classes—the day of the surgery and the day afterward. As an adjunct professor, I couldn't easily find coverage if I missed class and my students' education has always been important to me. I refused to let these temporary handicaps prevent me from teaching so I asked my cousin to accompany me to my two Friday freshmen composition courses. Once again, I was teaching through pain. However, this time was different. I had hope. I believed the endometriosis had been completely removed, and I'd be feeling like my old self again in no time. Even if I was experiencing the same pain, I understood that this was recovery. It had only been three days. It could go away. It would go away. It had to go away.

The doctor told me after the procedure that lesions covered my ovaries and bowel. In fact, they were so severe that my ovary and bowel had fused. I imagined festering sores sticking together, catching on each other like a fresh wound clings to a bandage. I'd see the images of reddish black patches—like cigarette burns to my reproductive organs. The explosion of red, thread-like veins swirling in nonsensical patterns and spots of dark-like punctuation marks signaling the end of healthy tissue. These pictures were chaos—nightmarish, abstract, visceral evidence of the crime scene inside my body, concealed within the the parts of me that should have been smooth, clean, biblical in their ability to create and sustain life; this was not the case.

It is a strange thing to experience joy at a diagnosis. I felt validated. I'll always remember sitting in the doctor's office one-week post-laparoscopy gazing at the shockingly clear and colorful photos of the lesions that decorated my left ovary and bowel. Like some kind of bizarre, abstract art, I admired these medical pictures of endometrial tissue obscuring my organs. These dark brown and pink bubbles were artifacts of my pain, and, according to my doctor, they'd been eradicated by the procedure. She promised I'd finally have relief.

Except that I didn't. At all. After this surgical procedure that finally identified and confirmed endometriosis, I was in just as severe, just as frequent pain as I was before the laparoscopy. How could this be? I was devastated all over again. I called the doctor, reported my lack of improvement, and returned, once again, to her office.

I was still experiencing the same endometriosis pain—sharp, radiating, extreme and mostly on my left side—that I had before the procedure when I went to the post-op appointment. The attractive blonde, middle-aged doctor with full cheeks and summer sky eyes frowned when I related the frequency and severity of my pain.

"You shouldn't be that uncomfortable. We removed the lesions and endometrial tissue." She gestured towards the images from the surgery as if they were proof. These pictures were evidence meant to discredit my claims. Although skeptical, she moved forward in the conversation as if I wasn't making it up, as if the endometriosis inside me was in fact still there, still causing me pain. Sitting there in that white room with the harsh fluorescent lighting, hands gripping the cold plastic cover of the examining table, I couldn't help but think of crab grass. Perhaps my endo was like these patches of weeds that will continue growing and setting seeds after they've been removed if you miss part of the stems when eradicating them. Maybe she missed a few stems or seeds.

She brought up the next step for treatment. I felt like throwing up. I was supposed to be done with all treatments. I was supposed to be better. In a voice made of sunshine and flowers and summer days at the beach, the doctor said, "Lupron injections." Perhaps she was just trying to make me feel better, but her cheery disposition made me want to scream. Smiling, she handed me a pamphlet detailing the use of the drug. I perused the material and nearly cried right there in her office once I'd finished reading.

Lupron shuts down the pituitary gland thus reducing the amount of estrogen a woman produces. This means that a woman's body is thrown into premature, artificial menopause.[2] I was horrified by the potential side effects: hot flashes, decreased sex drive, hair loss, bone loss, depression, anxiety, and more. What does this drug do to a women's fertility in the long term I wondered? Later on, I would read the testimonials of several women suffering from long term, devastating side effects of the drug, and the decision not to try Lupron was reinforced.

I recalled reading somewhere—maybe one of my online support groups—that most women who have laparoscopic surgeries for endometriosis ultimately have multiple surgeries—one surgery almost never resolves the issue permanently. Repeated surgeries can cause more damage, result in more scar tissue. I refused to do this again—ever.

---

2 "Lupron: National Women's Health Network." *National Women's Health Network* |, 24 Dec. 2020, https://nwhn.org/tag/lupron/

I left the appointment devastated. The entire drive home I wept. I wept and I wept and I wept until I had no tears left and I wasn't really weeping; just screeching. I remember that it was March and the day was gray. The trees were naked and lifeless from the harsh New England winter. Spring was around the corner, but it was hiding somewhere just out of reach.

It was during this car ride home that I started considering more extreme options: hysterectomy, pregnancy, expensive specialists in New York City. None of these solutions was ideal. I had already spent thousands of dollars on doctor's appointments, testing, and procedures with no results. I wasn't ready to have a baby; however, I did want to have a baby eventually so gutting myself wasn't a viable option either. I was at a loss.

Out of ideas and desperate for a permanent solution, I drove home, took a deep breath, and called my sister.

Jenny was five years younger than me. After we had outgrown the tag-a-long little sister/constantly irritated older sister dynamic, we became extremely close. Our relationship was one of support and almost maternal affection. I taught her how to write before she began school and read her stories on a regular basis. I helped with her homework in middle school. I was the one who took her to look at colleges when she was applying to schools in the middle of my parent's divorce. Of course I was also the one who got her drunk for the first time at my college apartment in Boston.

My sister and I were ying and yang, or Frank and Fred as we fondly dubbed each other at some point during our youth. We were contrary forces interconnected like winter and summer, the night and the day. I was the outgoing one, the extravert. She has always been fiercely private, introverted. Jenny loved astrology—she embodied the Gemini spirit in her curiosity and interest in new ideas which led to a discovery in her early twenties of holistic medicine.

I always felt the need to protect and guide my younger sister. So to reach out to her now for advice felt strange.

Her voice on the other end of the phone was a much needed salve. She mostly listened at first as I rattled off my spectrum of emotions followed by all the extreme solutions I'd come up with between the doctor's office and my house. When I had finished enumerating all the ways I could think of to put a definitive stop to my pain, she softly suggested a novel idea: Eastern medicine. If Western medicine had failed me so splendidly, then how much could it really hurt to try a completely new philosophy and practice? It was my turn to listen. She knew of an acupuncturist and naturopath that she'd recently seen who was helpful in treating her issues with acne. Jenny continued to sell me on the idea by mentioning that the worst case scenario was my pain didn't improve and we got a lunch date out of it. She mentioned a new Vietnamese place that had opened up in North Hampton. Not one to pass up an opportunity to spend an afternoon with my sister or to enjoy some good pho, I agreed to call the woman, set up an appointment, and make the two-hour drive from Connecticut to Western Massachusetts.

Although I had agreed to see a naturopath, I was still skeptical. Jenny was a recent convert to all things holistic, and, while she claimed she saw results, I had my doubts. Naturopath made me think of patchouli oil and anti-vaxxers and dread-locked hippies. But, then again, we've been conditioned as a society to subscribe to Western medicine and Western medicine only, and it had been failing me for years. Questions, like newly planted seeds, sprouted roots in my mind.

In a serendipitous turn of events, Greg and I went out for a friend's birthday dinner a few days after the conversation with Jenny. Sitting at the end of a long table, I struck up a conversation with the athletically built, dark-haired, middle-aged man sitting across from me. I had only spoken to Don a handful of times before and most of the chats were pleasant, but brief. On this night, over heaping trays of barbeque spare ribs, creamy macaroni and cheese, and mashed sweet potatoes dripping in butter, I came to know Don better and, consequently, learned more about Eastern medicine.

Apparently, Don was a licensed acupuncturist. He'd been a practitioner of Eastern medicine and holistic treatments since graduating from college in California in 2002 where he had completed a Masters of Science in Traditional Chinese Medicine. He regaled me with stories of women becoming pregnant after years of failed fertility treatments once they'd sought acupuncture as a path to pregnancy. He had impressive knowledge of endometriosis, more so then most of the Western doctors I'd encountered. He even directed me towards some online resources offering additional insight into Eastern treatments.

Between sips of ice water, Don explained my own condition to me in such an elegant and unusual way. My doctors had always spoken of endometriosis in clinical language laced with detached tones and medical jargon. Don told me, "Endometriosis is usually defined as "blood stagnation" with several root causes such as "Qi Stagnation" or "Yang Deficiency." Of course these were strange, new terms but they had an almost beautiful, poetic quality to them. Perhaps it was the soothing voice of a licensed acupuncturist vs. a doctor, but Don had piqued my interest, and I asked him to continue. "One must treat the root cause and also treat the branch symptom." He painted a picture of my chronic illness as if it was a plant that simply needed to be tended with care. Continuing, "Acupuncture and Auriciular techniques are usually used to reduce pain, inflammation, and move blood, as well as hormones. Herbal formulas are similarly targeted towards addressing both root and branch, specifically stopping bleeding and warming to promote circulation and reduce pain." I was fascinated.

I remember taking in the smell of smoky air, the kind that sticks to your clothes long after you've gone home. Burst of laughter, lively conversation, and the clinking of silverware against plates provided the soundtrack to this moment. This man offered solutions that went completely against the conventional attitude towards sickness and healing. Don the raconteur and holistic guru had crafted a seductive tale of hope and healing. Was this guy a snake oil salesman or did he actually have a way to treat my disease that wouldn't put me into more medical debt or menopause at thirty?

The phone conversation with Jenny coupled with the auspicious dinner discussion led to an epiphany: there just might be another way to manage my pain and treat endometriosis. I just had to be willing to take a chance. And you know what? I was.

7

EASTERN MEDICINE

Rooms filled with clouds of incense. Enya songs playing softly in the background of an office filled with futons and Bonsai plants and tiny water fountains. Doctors who aren't really doctors wearing white linen pants and flip flops and drinking tea as they prescribe meditation and yoga to treat visceral ailments and scoff at modern medicine. These were the images that "Eastern medicine" conjured before I encountered it. I was, like most of the folks I know, a skeptic. However, when you've followed the conventional path towards healing and you see few results, you tend to become more amenable to formally laughable solutions.

I scheduled an appointment with a naturopath named Elizabeth for an early Saturday morning a few weeks after the conversations with Jenny and Don. To arrive at the office in Massachusetts punctually, I needed to leave by six a.m. The morning announced itself in bursts of gold, orange, and blue—a match just before it burns out. There was no traffic on 84 that early in the day. A few tractor trailers cruised in the center lane until I approached Hartford. The radio played loudly and a cold wind snapped through the slightly open window. I tried not to think about the pain pulsing in my abdomen or the the anxiety inextricably connected with the unknown. *Would this appointment be a waste of time? Is it worth driving two hours when I could be laying in bed with my heating pad?*

Even with my GPS, I still managed to get lost on my way to the naturopath's office. A plain storefront in a small plaza, the office was surrounded by Enterprise Rent-A-Car, a CVS, gas station, and D'Angelo's Grilled Sandwiches. *A peculiar place for a healing oasis* I thought to myself. I had imagined a contemporary-styled building or big Victorian house nestled among lush flowering shrubs and sprawling oak trees. This location was simple, cosmopolitan, congested. A shopping plaza on a busy six-lane road. Angry horns punctuated the morning air as traffic lights winked and heavy traffic roared. *Not the sanctuary I pictured.*

Feeling uncertain and a little nervous, I exited the car and went inside the office. No one was around. The front desk was empty, the waiting area quiet with several vacant chairs. I cleared my throat in the hope that someone might hear. A pretty woman much younger than I had envisioned, she couldn't have been more than mid-thirties, appeared smiling from a hallway behind the desk. She wore her brown hair in a ponytail and a white lab coat over professional clothing—a blouse and slacks. Her greeting was unexpectedly affable, like an invitation lost in the mail when it suddenly arrives. And she was noticeably pregnant.

"Can I get you a cup of tea?" She offered before taking me into a room down the hallway.

I declined and thanked her as we entered a dimly lit room with a bed in the center—more massage parlor than doctor's office. We sat opposite of each other in a pair of comfortable, darkly upholstered chairs. Elizabeth began the appointment by asking me about my symptoms. However, unlike traditional doctors, this naturopath wasn't simply interested in my ailments. She wanted to hear my story. For the first time in my life, a medical professional wanted to hear every detail.

"Tell me everything. From the beginning. Don't leave anything out, even if it doesn't feel relevant."

So I did. The pain narrative I had composed over the last several years finally had an audience. Elizabeth listened intently, taking notes in a little book as I went. She nodded occasionally, smiled encouragingly, and interjected with a few questions here and there. The very act of telling my story had an almost therapeutic effect. At last, a medical professional cared enough to sit with me and hear me talk about the episodes of pain unaffected by medication or surgery, the unending series of pointless doctor's visits, and the tests that provided no additional insights into my condition.

The second surprise of the visit came next. After a few related follow-up questions, Elizabeth asked if it would be alright if she felt my wrist. She explained that she was performing a pulse diagnosis. Placing three fingers over the radial artery in the wrist, she was looking for pulse length, depth, and quality as these pulse attributes would reveal information about my overall health. Short or long pulse length indicates strength and balance of blood and energy flow. For example, a short, forceful pulse reflects a stagnant condition which means the blood isn't flowing well because of blockages. The pulse depth reveals pathological conditions. In other words, pulse felt at the superficial level indicates an exterior illness like a cold whereas deep pulse reflects internal conditions and the state of the organs. The third attribute she was examining was the pulse quality. These qualities can range from choppy, rough pulse with uneven flow to slippery. Ascertaining the quality of the pulse would allow her to determine heat vs. dampness, conditions that are indicative of energy more than actual temperature.[3]

She read my pulse like a mystic reading a palm, but instead of looking into a nebulous future and making tenuous claims, she offered shockingly concrete interpretations of my present state: My general health was good, however, something was off in my body. I was experiencing pain at that exact moment. She even told me the precise location of this pain. She had more revelatory insights with her next test: tongue diagnosis.

Sans depressor and equipped with nothing more than a pair of brightly shining eyes, Elizabeth studied my tongue like it was a map and she was the cartographer able to decipher its legend. She articulated the topography of my pain indicated by the size, shape, color and coating of my tongue. Using these attributes as if they were faded lines and ancient symbols, she described my general health, diet, and lifestyle. For example, a thicker coating indicates sickness. A pale color suggests cold and some kind of deficiency in the body.[4] These clues told her that while my diet was mostly healthy (it was), I ate quite a bit of dairy (guilty). She thought I might be experiencing an unhealthy amount of stress (yes!), and, of course, there was a deficiency in my body (endometriosis).

In less than a half hour, this naturopath had a more intimate grasp of my health than any previous doctor I had seen. The initial diagnostic process was followed by a series of prescriptive actions:

---

3 Dubowsky, Jennifer. "Pulse Power: Understanding Pulses in Chinese Medicine." *Qi Blog*, 16 Oct. 2014, https://qiblog.emperors.edu/2014/09/pulse-power-understanding-tcm-pulse-diagnosis/

4 http://www.acupuncture.edu/2016/09/28/understanding-tongue-diagnosis-in-chinese-medicine/

first, a cocktail of herbs that I should begin taking regularly. Secondly, dietary changes including limiting dairy and gluten and eating more cooked and warm foods. Lastly, acupuncture.

The treatment she administered that day came in the form of a series of tiny needles placed in different points throughout my body. Lying on a comfortable bed in the center of the room, Elizabeth placed the needles in my ankles, legs, and arms. A warm water bottle and heated blanket were then placed on my abdomen. She played classical music on her iPhone and instructed me to relax for the next twenty minutes. I must have fallen asleep because the next thing I remember is waking up in the dimly lit room to a knock on the door.

"How do you feel?"

I was still uncomfortable, but the pain had dulled somewhat. It was, after all, only the first appointment. Experience had made me realistic; I wasn't expecting a miracle.

I spent a full hour in Elizabeth's office for this first appointment. When I walked to the counter to give her payment, I expected an astronomical bill that I'd have to break up into smaller payments since my Connecticut insurance would certainly not cover any of this appointment. Instead, she asked me for seventy-five dollars—a shockingly reasonable amount for the services rendered. The subsequent visits would cost fifty dollars. This amount was comparable to the co-pays I paid at the other doctor's offices, however, that was with insurance, and I'd often receive additional bills for tests or services after the visit. This visit was covered, out-of-pocket, with that one-time payment.

Outside of the office, the morning was bright. The sky was a blank cerulean canvas. The sounds of traffic filled the air as I made my way to the car. No trees, no water fountains, no Enya music, but perhaps this was an oasis after all.

8

AN ALTERNATIVE APPROACH

Did chronic pain exist in Ancient Egypt or during the Middle Ages? Did Renaissance women suffer from endometriosis? I imagine women in tight bodices and layers of long skirts doubled over in pain. Before the advent of modern medicine, how did women treat their pain? For centuries, apothecaries provided medicines—mostly herbs, plants, and oils. In 3rd Century China, apothecaries derived medicines from grasses and roots, and some of these early treatments eventually introduced ephedrine. As early as the beginning of the 20th century, Western doctors recognized what would eventually be known as endometriosis.

In 1903, Mayer (14) published a description of what could be the first case of secondary endometriosis. During a re-laparotomy for severe pelvic pains after a uterine ventrofixation, he found epithelial glands around the silk ligatures. To justify their presence, he elaborated his theory of epithelial heterotopy, considering it a sort of healing process; for him, adenomyomas were examples of "epithelial invasion of inflammatory infiltrated tissue" (14). [5]

According to this text, Western doctors have known about the existence of endometriosis for over a hundred years and yet the disease is barely understood. There is no definitive cause or proven cure or treatment. Doctors proscribe birth control pills, Lupron injections, surgeries, and hysterectomies to manage this chronic illness. How is it that after a century the medical industry's solution is to slice into us, mutilate us further, gut us like farm animals? Or, perhaps less extreme, yet no less grotesque, render us infertile, stop ovulation, induce premature menopause? If we don't understand it and we can't control, let's eradicate it. Is this simply a different form of diagnosing depressed women as hysterics and prescribing rest and isolation?

Traditional Chinese Medicine, on the other hand, closely examines endometriosis and offers a comprehensive portrait of female health. This nuanced look considers everything from quality of menstrual blood to liver health and the presence of stress in a woman's life.[6]

ACUPUNCTURE

Acupuncture became a ritual like taking a shower in the morning or reading news headlines over breakfast. I drove two hours to visit

5   *Define_me*, https://www.fertstert.org/article/S0015-0282(10)00980-5/pdf#:~:text=In%201903%2C%20Mayer%20(14),glands%20around%20the%20silk%20ligatures

6   Pcom. "TCM to Treat Endometriosis Symptoms." *Pacific College*, 8 Jan. 2019, https://www.pacificcollege.edu/news/blog/2015/02/26/tcm-to-treat-endometriosis-symptoms

Elizabeth about once a month. I continued the treatments along with the herbal supplements she suggested and other holistic practices such as castor oil packs and dietary changes. I experienced relief from these acupuncture sessions with Elizabeth, but it was her guidance and help in curating a list of herbs as well as refining my diet that was perhaps most impactful in treating endo.

As months slipped away and holistic treatments became lifestyle choices, my pain noticeably diminished. For a year or so, I continued to make the trip for early morning sessions with Elizabeth. She continued pricking me with tiny needles as I lay in a heated bed while classical music and spa sounds played from her iPhone. Eventually, the trip became too much, and as I began to feel better and regain a sense of control over my body once more, acupuncture became more occasional than regular.

TEA

I've never been a coffee person. While I love the smell of the brew percolating in the morning, I've always preferred the taste of a hot cup of tea. In high school, I'd enjoy a mug of Earl Grey with milk and honey as I did my homework after school. As a college student, it was a cup of black tea, usually Lipton, with cookies at the end of the day as I watched ABC melodramas to decompress. Tea wasn't just a satisfying beverage I drank to quench a thirst; it was a drink of comfort, a safety blanket, the taste of home when I was stressed or sad or overwhelmed. And as the years passed, tea became a salve, an elixir of sorts that did more than ease my mind, it alleviated my physical pain. Although tea has always been an important part of my life, it wasn't until 2016 that it became essential. More than simply my preferred caffeinated beverage, green and herbal teas have proven to be helpful in reducing endometriosis pain.

The switch to green tea in my early twenties was strictly pragmatic: green tea, I'd read, was healthier. I educated myself about matcha, a special form of powdered green tea. Traditional green tea is prepared by steeping tea bags filled with green tea leaves in hot water. Matcha green tea contains the actual tea leaves which have been ground into a powder substance. The process of creating matcha is unique in that the tea plants are covered with shade clothes several weeks before harvesting in order to promote flavor and texture. [7] Because the tea leaves themselves are ingested when drinking this beverage, the concentration of antioxidants is greater than traditional green tea. Furthermore, the caffeine-boost from this drink is, in my opinion, better than a cup of coffee or other forms of tea.

Herbal tea blends containing certain flowers, roots, and herbs have proven beneficial specifically in mitigating my endometriosis pain. Certain plants effectively balance female hormones, and, I learned, in assuaging chronic pain. Regular consumption of herbal tea blends containing chaste berry (or Vitex) and raspberry leaf are the most helpful.

Chaste berry, also known as vitex, is a small, brown berry that has been used by naturopaths and holistic practitioners to ease PMS symptoms and boost fertility. One of my favorite herbal tea blends is a red tea that proclaims to boost skin health. It is a rooibos and chamomile tea that contains an amalgamation of chaste berry and various other berries, flowers, and roots such as hibiscus, red clover, burdock root, and orange peel. The beverage has a pomegranate essence and is as delicious as it is powerful. I try to drink two cups of this tea daily and have found that it reduces pain frequency.

Raspberry leaf is commonly known to balance female hormones and promote fertility and thus is commonly referred to as the woman's herb. Some research supports the claim that the leaves help relieve premenstrual symptoms (PMS) such as cramping, vomiting, nausea,

---

7   Cynthia Sass, MPH. "Matcha: Benefits, Nutrition, and Risks." *Health*, Health, 20 Sept. 2022, https://www.health.com/nutrition/what-is-matcha

and diarrhea. The leaves contain fragarine, a plant compound that helps tone and tighten muscles in the pelvic area, which may reduce the menstrual cramping caused by the spasms of these muscles.[8] It seems logical then that the painful spasms associated with endometriosis could also be improved with regular consumption of the leaves.

In my research into Eastern medicine, I also came across an article which suggested drinking primarily hot or room temperature beverages versus cold ones can help the body combat endometriosis. I switched to drinking hot mugs of water in place of cold filtered or bottled water. In Chinese Medicine, an excess of cold fluids can contribute to slow digestion and stomach heat which can impact the female body in a negative way. [9]

Dorothee, a silver-haired woman who owns a winery in upstate New York, met me for a cup of tea at a café in Connecticut one afternoon not long after reaching out via email. She had read an article I wrote about the impact drinking tea has had on my endometriosis pain. As it turns out, Dorothee was also a researcher looking into the way cheek cells respond to plant pigments, and my claims fit her research perfectly.

Dorothee has spent thirty years researching plant pigments and how they can be used to diagnose endometriosis through saliva. She was very interested in discussing my experience with alternative methods of managing endometriosis pain. Dorothee explained to me that the cheek cells respond differently to certain plant pigments like quercetin (found in oak) and certain anthocyanins found in berries.

---

8   Goodson, Amy. "Red Raspberry Leaf Tea: Pregnancy, Benefits and Side Effects." *Healthline*, Healthline Media, 30 July 2018, https://www.healthline.com/nutrition/red-raspberry-leaf-tea#benefits

9   "Avoiding Cold Beverages – Why?" *Nis Chinese Medical Center*, https://www.drboni.com/?p=496

In fact, she said, skin cells stain differently for women suffering from endometriosis. She also told me that she hopes to develop a simple, easy-to-use test that can allow women to track when endometriosis flares up.

HERBAL SUPPLEMENTS & VITAMINS

A team of acupuncturists and herbalists have explored the correlation between Chinese herbs and the treatment of endometriosis citing a scientific study that was performed several decades ago. Although this particular study is over forty years old, the findings are interesting, relevant, and substantiate the experiences and claims of many endo warriors pursuing holistic paths. They write,

> In 1980 researchers at the Hospital of Obstetrics and Gynecology of the Shanghai First Medical College conducted a clinical trial using Chinese herbs to treat endometriosis. 156 endometriosis sufferers were divided into three groups and then given an herbal formula that addressed blood stagnation as well as their underlying condition. According to the report, 82% of the women* saw their symptoms mostly or entirely alleviated, while 18% of the women* had either no effect or any beneficial effect was very short term and was lost when the herbs were discontinued.
>
> To me what this research means is that Chinese herbs are effective in the treatment of endometriosis but only if a full diagnosis is made and if treatment is specifically tailored to fit the patient's individual pattern.[10]

---

10 "Endometriosis – A Chinese Medicine Approach." *The Yinova Center*, 28 Sept. 2021, https://www.yinovacenter.com/blog/endometriosis-a-chinese-medicine-approach/

Eighty-two percent of the women in this study saw their endometriosis symptoms mostly or entirely alleviated with Chinese herbs. That is significant! While this is a relatively small sample of women and the study is from the early 1980s, the conclusions are important. They support the experience of many endo-warriors who have turned to holistic treatments for relief.

Spirulina is one herbal supplement that I've integrated into my daily routine. This superfood contains high levels of vitamins, protein, antioxidants, and inflammation-fighting properties.[11] I believe that it is these inflammation-fighting qualities that make Spirulina worthwhile for endo-sufferers. These blue-green algae need to stay refrigerated and the tablets have a strong, fishy flavor, however, I combat this offensive taste by reverting back to my childhood and holding my breath as I ingest them. It's not the most mature approach, but it works!

Cramp Bark Plus is one of the best supplements I found for alleviating endometriosis symptoms. A description of the herbal cocktail and its value in Eastern medicine is as follows:

> Crampbark (Viburnum opulis) is a Native American remedy with warming and antispasmodic actions used for menstrual cramps. This herb is combined with warm, blood-vitalizing herbs that also help to relieve menstrual pains. Cramp Bark Plus is based on formulas for uterine cramping, Cinnamon and Persica Combination, Achyranthes Combination, and To Jing Wan. Also included in the formula are herbs that assist circulation of Qi and moisture, leonurus (yi mu cao), and vladimiria souliei (mu

---

11 "Spirulina: Dosage, Eye Health, Oral Health, and More." *Medical News Today*, MediLexicon International, https://www.medicalnewstoday.com/articles/324027.php

xiang). Zedoaria (e zhu) and sparganium (san leng) are traditionally used to reduce fibroids and cysts. In conformity with traditional Chinese practice, the herbs have been soaked in wine, and then dried, prior to tableting. This process enhances the warming and blood vitalizing properties of Cramp Bark Plus.[12]

I took several pills daily as part of my regimen, and they curbed endo pain effectively.

One of the numerous doctors of Western Medicine I encountered on my path to healing explained that most women who suffer from endometriosis also suffer from low vitamin D. This finding was echoed by Elizabeth during our initial meeting. I added a vitamin D supplement to my regimen when I learned my levels were indeed low after getting blood work done.

My carefully curated list of supplements and teas was derived from a combination of independent research, recommendations from a naturopath, and, honestly, trial and error. Because each case of endometriosis is as different as the woman who suffers from the disease, each ultimately beneficial cocktail of herbs will have to be determined by the woman herself, with or without guidance from a naturopath or physician. These holistic approaches can also be effective for women adhering to a more conventional treatment plan.

EXERCISE

The logic behind this holistic solution is obvious; however, let's be honest: sometimes exercise is hard, especially if you are in the middle of a flare. I mean, how often do you think *I'm feeling crappy today, I should workout.* If you do, you are superhuman and please share your secret with me. When I'm feel especially motivated (on occasion), I

---

12 "Health Concerns Cramp Bark plus - 90 Capsules." *Lhasa OMS*, https://www.lhasaoms.com/health-concerns-cramp-bark-plus

do make it to the gym in the middle of a flare. I know that running on the treadmill when I am experiencing an episode can make the pain worse; however, I've learned to listen to my body. When she's whispering *slow down, easy* I obey; I don't push her. If the whisper becomes a whimper, I stop, I switch from jog to walk. If she starts yelling at me, I take a break from the treadmill, walk to the locker room, and focus on breathing to calm her down.

In theory, cardio and aerobic workouts not only benefit general health and increase fitness, but, according to Chinese medicine, they reduce symptoms of endometriosis. The Pacific College of Oriental Medicine writes in *Traditional Chinese Medicine to Treat Endometriosis Symptoms* that "each life force has an innate energy flowing throughout its form. This is called "qi" and qi is also believed to move the blood. Stagnant qi is associated with liver depression. The liver is so intimately associated with the menstrual cycle, liver depression and stagnant qi in women almost always manifests as some menstrual-related problem. Exercise can also speed up a sluggish metabolism and increase production of qi and blood. Aerobic exercise from twenty to thirty minutes every other day increases circulation and body temperature, and aids digestion, appetite, mood, energy and sleep. Exercise greatly reduces the severity of any endometriosis symptom or symptom associated with stagnant qi and blood stasis."[13] In other words, it is recommended that a person seeking healing through alternative treatments should be sure to include an exercise regime of some kind.

Exercise was already a part of my lifestyle. Even before pursuing Eastern medicine and a holistic path, I went to the gym around three times a week. Cardio—primarily running on a treadmill for around

---

13 Pcom. "TCM to Treat Endometriosis Symptoms." *Pacific College*, 8 Jan. 2019, https://www.pacificcollege.edu/news/blog/2015/02/26/ tcm-to-treat-endometriosis-symptoms

twenty-five minutes—was the the crux of my workout routine. However, I'd often experience bursts of endo pain mid-run, sometimes so painful that I'd have to instantly stop, leave the machine, and rush into the ladies' locker room to crouch down into a squatting position. If other women were around, I'd pretend I was stretching or doing some sort of deep-breathing exercise. In reality, I was struggling to keep from crying and trying to maintain an even breath. If the pain was too overwhelming, I'd cut my workout short for the day and drive home well over the speed limit. On better days, I'd wait five minutes or so for the pain to subside, and I'd return to the same treadmill. I'd ease back into the run, walking slowly through the pain until it was mostly gone. I always did feel better afterwards, if I was able to stick it out. I'm not sure if this effect was physical like the tenants of Chinese Medicine claim, or if I was simply high off the endorphins released from the activity. Either way, I did find relief even if only for a little while.

I've also learned to amend my workout routine as my pain dictates. Although I am fortunate enough that endo pain is infrequent now, I still have the occasional bad days. When these pain days conflict with my cardio schedule, I adjust accordingly. For example, I recently had an endo flare which caused painsomnia and left me exhausted and in mild discomfort in the morning. It was supposed to be a cardio gym day, but I assessed my body and gave myself grace. I anticipated a continued flare if I attempted to do my usual workout so instead I opted to stay home and focus on a light glute and ab routine. It was not as rigorous as a cardio day, but I avoided triggering any additional endo pain and still burned some calories which left me feeling good despite the disrupted sleep cycle of the previous night.

ESSENTIAL OIL

In addition to endometriosis, I also suffer from ovarian cysts and endometriomas, or cystic masses in the ovaries filled with tar-like fluid that give them their moniker "chocolate cysts." Such a benign moniker is ill-fitting as these endometriomas have caused pain so severe I've vomited from it. The most recent flare-up of these little chocolate nightmares was so severe I ended up in the doctor's office getting an ultrasound to confirm that was actually what was going on.

After complaining about the pain from with these ovarian cysts to my friend and writing buddy, Hayley, she recommended that I try taking a tablespoon of extra virgin olive oil each day. Hayley has also experienced frustration with ovarian cysts and endometriosis and was someone whose advice I greatly respected when it came to managing these things. In fact, it was Hayley who suggested a delicious coconut milk yogurt substitute when I was struggling to eliminate dairy from my diet. If she could convince me to stop eating regular yogurts, which I had done every day for basically my entire life, then she probably had some other useful insights. Adding a tablespoon of olive oil first thing in the morning before breakfast or beverages proved to be an invaluable addition to my regimen. I might even say that a shot of olive oil a day, keeps the endometriomas away!

My sister Jenny has also contributed some very helpful essential oil blends to my routine. She blended evening primrose oil, clary sage, frankincense, lavender, neroli, and ylang ylang and put them in a roller bottle. Upon her instruction, I massage the oils over my neck (thyroid) and along my lower back (over kidneys) each morning and night. I've noticed that after several months of this ritual my periods are less painful and significantly lighter. I don't know for sure if this is a direct result of the essential oils or something else, however, it is the only new component of my holistic regimen.

Additionally, massaging thyme oil over the abdomen provides great relief from cramps. Thyme essential oil is known for analgesic and antispasmodic effects which likely help with menstrual pain.

CASTOR OIL PACKS & CBD

One approach to pain management that can be both soothing mid-flare and preventative is the castor oil pack.

The bottle of pale yellow liquid is sticky to the touch—some residual oil must have dripped the last time I used it. I twist off the white bottle cap, my fingers now coated in gooey liquid that smells of castor beans. Taking two paper towels which are folded in half to create a square, sufficiently thick cloth, I pour a small amount of castor oil directly on the makeshift applicator. The pale yellow oil pools on the cloth, only somewhat absorbed. It stretches out but retains a circular shape—like a sun against a white, clouded sky. Carefully holding the paper towel in my hand, I make my way to the living room couch. The heating pad is already plugged in and warming up. I pull up my sweatshirt, pull down my pants and underwear so that I can place the pack on my bare skin. Quickly, I flip the paper towel so that the wet, oiled side is directly on the left side of my abdomen and pelvic area, exactly where the pain is beginning to cramp and stab uncomfortably. It is cold where it hits flesh, and I even feel a quick tingling sensation as the oil sets into place. Sometimes the oil will leak onto my clothing or other areas so it helps to have an extra cloth or paper towel nearby to wipe any spillage. Once the pack is in place, I put the heating pad on top of it and let it work its magic. I pull my shirt back down over the heating pad, grab the TV remote, and find whatever show I am enjoying on Netflix.

Within about fifteen or twenty minutes, the pain begins to abate. I'll leave the pack on though for at least forty-five minutes or for a full episode of a TV show. Doing this about three or four times per week can be preventative, but applying a castor pack mid or early into a pain flare can also be very effective. The cool prick of the oil seeping into my pores paired with the mollifying heat provides relief that Tylenol or Advil or Aleve fails to do. This treatment was suggested by my naturopath as a means of reducing pain and inflammation (which endometriosis is) as well as shrinking any growths like uterine fibroids or cysts.

Castor oil is a vegetable oil that is extracted from castor bean seeds. Having multiple uses, this oil has been used for thousands of years for everything from practical purposes to medicinal. Most commonly known for its use as a laxative, it can be used as a natural and fast-acting laxative to relieve constipation. Rich in ricinoleic acid, a monounsaturated fatty acid, castor oil can be used to moisturize skin. Anti-inflammatory properties have been shown in some studies to reduce inflammation and pain when used topically.[14]

From the endometriosis support groups and networks that I follow, I've learned that some endo warriors have also experienced relief using CBD oil. Cannabidiol oil, more commonly referred to as CBD, is quickly becoming a go-to for many people with chronic pain and other issues like anxiety and depression. In a 2021 article published on *Healthline*, Jessica Timmons writes,

> Your body has what's known as the endocannabinoid system (ECS). It's made up of **endocannabinoids:** These molecules are made by the human body. They're similar to the cannabinoids found in cannabis. These compounds work on receptors found throughout the body. **Receptors:** CB1 receptors are primarily found in the central nervous system. CB2 receptors are typically found in the peripheral nervous system. **Enzymes.** Enzymes break down endocannabinoids after they've carried out their functions. Some cannabinoids, like THC, are known to bind to ECS receptors. Other cannabinoids, like CBD, interact with the system in a different way. One theory is that CBD slows the

---

14 Kubala, Jillian. "Castor Oil: 4 Benefits and Uses." *Healthline*, Healthline Media, 28 Jan. 2022, https://www.healthline.com/nutrition/castor-oil #TOC_TITLE_HDR_5

process of breaking endocannabinoids down, allowing them to remain effective for longer.[15]

Furthermore, she says, "Most significantly for people with endometriosis, research from 2017 suggests that the ECS interacts with many of the pain-associated mechanisms of this condition. Researchers say that influencing the ECS might be a good strategy for relieving pain." My personal experience with CBD has consisted of popping a gummy or two if my anxiety sets in, however, I am open to trying it for endometriosis pain when and if I need it.

HEAT

When you have endometriosis, heating pads are life. Heating pads are everything. In the hottest days of summer, you can find me curled up with my heating pad, temperature on maximum. I might be dripping in sweat, but that pad better be hot as Hades. If your skin isn't bright pink on the verge of a first-degree burn, do you even use it correctly? In all seriousness, I've always found the hotter the heating pad, the more soothing it is.

I've also discovered that car seat warmers can also be very effective in relieving endo pain. The front seat of my husband's truck has seat warmers that are all-encompassing and seem to reach a blissful level of hot—beyond the normal heat I've become accustomed to with the pad. I will, on occasion, find an excuse to go for a ride in his truck simply to enjoy sitting as a passenger. The heat on my bottom and back is immeasurably soothing.

---

15 Timmons, Jessica. "4 Best CBD Products for Endometriosis Pain 2022." *Healthline*, Healthline Media, 14 July 2022, https://www.healthline.com/health/cbd-for-endometriosis#endocannabinoid-system

TENS MACHINE

Greg came home from work one night bearing a gift. Not the kind of guy who surprises me with sweet, just-because tokens of his affection, I was caught off guard. He was excited handing me a small, unwrapped package. A white, round objected with what looked like ear buds attached to it, like a futuristic iPod, the TENS Machine immediately piqued my interest. I'd read about how Transcutaneous Electrical Nerve Stimulation (TENS) may reduce endometriosis related pain by blocking the pain signal from reaching the brain, increasing blood circulation to targeted areas and stimulating the body's natural painkillers. The little ear bud-like wires attached to two oddly shaped pads that had a sticky adhesive substance. The device itself had a button which indicated more or less power intensity, much like a volume button.

A few days after he got the device, I had a minor flare up so I decided to give it a try. Accustomed to the soothing, comforting warmth of my heating pad, it was a different feeling to apply a cold plastic device to the left side of my abdomen. The pulses that come from the TENS machine are strange, like a mild pinching sensation, but the warm vibrations seemed to untangle the pain knots forming in my abdomen and pelvis. I adjusted the intensity of the electrical modes until it was just right—not too powerful but not too gentle either. It seemed to provide some relief although, oddly enough, I missed the warmth of my heating pad which had been my traditional source of comfort and relief for so long.

ALCOHOL & LIVER HEALTH

From September to December 2013, I did not have a single drink of an alcoholic beverage. I replaced Vodka cranberries and glasses of white wine with a mug of hot water with lemon or a cup of tea. I remained social, still frequented bars and social gatherings that revolved around drinking, and no one judged my sudden switch from cocktails to sober drinks. And I rather enjoyed waking up on Sunday mornings feeling refreshed.

Until I gave up imbibing, I did not realize the physical impact alcohol had on my body. Not only did I sleep better and have more energy overall, I suspected that my endometriosis was more manageable without the boozy trigger. Once I cut back on drinking, I noticed that I would have substantial flare-ups the day after a particularly drunk evening. For all these reasons, even after I gave up teetotaling, I cut way back on alcohol consumption. I went from drinking every weekend and occasionally during the week, to easily going without drinks for weeks or months at a time.

This theory was put to the test on a girls' trip to Nashville, Tennessee. I spent the last day of our four-day trip in bed, in the hotel room, curled into a fetal position while pain flared up with a rage I hadn't experienced in some time. Clearly, my body was pissed off. Endometriosis woke with a start, aroused and enraged by all kinds of alcoholic beverages—sugary cocktails, shots of tequila, mixed drinks with cute names—and threw quite a temper tantrum. It was certainly compounded by the not-so-endo-friendly meals we'd eaten the entire time we were in Nashville: rich, buttery, carb-filled breakfasts and slow-cooked, spicy, BBQ-lathered meats for lunches and dinner—the cuisine in Nashville was positively divine; my digestive system and lingering endometriosis clearly disagreed. What resulted was frequent trips to the bathroom, horrific cramping and an epic flare-up that kept me in the hotel on the last day of our trip. I missed The Grand Ole Opry!

In Chinese medicine, there is a connection between liver health and endometriosis. According to Pacific College of Health and Science, "In Chinese medicine, the uterus and the liver are closely related. The liver maintains patency or free flow of the qi or vital energy of the body. The liver, spleen, and kidney channels run through the pelvis and all can effect menstruation. If any of these channels is blocked, congested or deficient, this will usually manifest in women as some sort of menstrual problem."[16] The connection between liver health and endometriosis seemed quite logical once I had reduced alcohol consumption.

A holistic practice specializing in fertility and endometriosis adds this about the connection between liver health and endometriosis: "As endometrial tissue is affected by estrogen it is helpful to avoid a condition called "estrogen dominance." The liver is responsible for metabolizing excess estrogen and so supporting good liver function is an important part of a holistic strategy to treat endometriosis. Because of this, we advise our patients with endometriosis to limit their alcohol consumption and avoid caffeine. You may also want to discuss with your practitioner ways of using liver-supporting herbs such as dandelion, milk thistle, and burdock root as part of your herbal regimen.[17]

Burdock root and dandelion are two herbs that have substantial benefits to liver health, and, therefore, endometriosis relief. Both are commonly found in herbal teas as well as in pill or extract form. The root of the burdock plant, which is native to North Asia and Europe, has nutrients such as antioxidants and inulin which are known to aid in digestion and reduce inflammation. Similarly, dandelion contains antioxidants and can help flight inflammation. Animal studies have found that dandelion has a protective effect on liver tissue in the presence of toxic substances and stress.[18]

---

16 https://www.pacificcollege.edu/news/blog/2015/02/26/tcm-to-treat-endometriosis-symptoms

17 "Endometriosis – A Chinese Medicine Approach." *The Yinova Center*, 28 Sept. 2021, https://www.yinovacenter.com/blog/endometriosis-a-chinese-medicine-approach/

18 Link, Rachael. "Dandelion: Health Benefits and Side Effects." *Healthline*, Healthline Media, 4 Jan. 2022, https://www.healthline.com/nutrition/dandelion-benefits#TOC_TITLE_HDR_8

Blending different herbs such as burdock root and dandelion in delicious teas or simply taking them in supplement form has immense health benefits for those trying to boost liver health. The connection between liver health and endometriosis is logical—the liver purges the body of excess estrogen and toxins. Estrogen promotes endo growth. A holistic combination of less booze and more herbs that promote healthy livers is just one aspect of a rigorous alternative regime.

Since I tend not to experience any pain relief from over the counter medicine or pain relievers, I will sometimes take a shot of milk thistle in the middle of a painful episode. I typically see an end to the flare-up within a half hour of taking the milk thistle.

For this reason, not only did I reduce consumption of alcohol, I began taking milk thistle. Milk thistle rids the liver of toxins and promotes overall liver health. Silymarin is the primary component of milk thistle seeds, and it is thought to alleviate symptoms of liver disorders such as hepatitis and cirrhosis.[19] Available in capsule, powder, or extract form, I drank milk thistle as an extract diluted with water. Filling the dropper with the solution, I'd add it to about two ounces of water, and chug it as if it was a shot of liquor. I'd try to drink this solution two to four times a day.

I enjoy a glass of wine now and then or a mixed drink or several when out with friends. And I still every so often like to tie one on; however, I don't get wasted every weekend. In fact, you can sometimes find me at the bar enjoying a steaming cup of green tea.

---

19 "Milk Thistle." *National Center for Complementary and Integrative Health*, U.S. Department of Health and Human Services, https://nccih.nih.gov/health/milkthistle/ataglance.htm

9

DISORDERED EATING,
BODY IMAGE & GLUTEN-FREE DIET

We live in a world where girls are taught from a young age to hate their bodies. The introduction of social media into adolescent lives has only made this self-loathing more profound. As a teacher, I've read so many papers over the course of the last few years about young women and their various eating disorders, issues which have only been amplified by Instagram and TikTok and the multifarious media images of "beautiful" women. I grieve for these young women—and men—who find themselves overwhelmed with the desire to emulate these edited and filtered and unrealistic bodies. And I am grateful. Grateful that as a young, self-conscious teenager with my own set of unhealthy eating habits and terrible body-image there was no social media to reinforce these ideals and to lead me down a darker path than the one that already beckoned.

My relationship with food has always been complex. Growing up, I could eat anything I wanted without fear of gaining weight, and I was raised in a household that valued hearty meals followed by my mother's homemade desserts. I was raised on breaded pork chops, creamy chicken dishes, and apple turnovers with vanilla ice-cream. These were the days before farm-to-table dishes, quinoa, and organic produce. I'm pretty sure kale hadn't even been invented yet. After school snacks were bags of potato chips, Oreos, freshly baked chocolate chip cookies, bowls of sugary cereal. This was the '90s and people weren't talking about GMO's or asking questions about ingredients. I'm pretty sure parents grocery shopping didn't even notice there were labels on products. Throw it in the cart, kid, and let's get out of here.

But when I turned fifteen, puberty had finished molding soft, womanly curves and the voracious appetite and extra calories essential to the sculpting process were no longer necessary. In a relatively short period of time, I went from wearing a size zero to a six. The pale, flat sheet of my belly began to ripple with new layers of skin that billowed over the top of my pants.

I obsessed about my weight. I pushed myself to work out—running on a treadmill for as long as I could without cramping, a few stretches, and some weight lifting—to no results. I had difficulty motivating myself to exercise; I despised it. I was a high school girl whose social activities revolved around Starbuck's hangouts, late night ice-cream runs, and drinking beer or whatever cheap liquor we could get our hands on. The number on the scale was steadily rising, but I was a teenager who wore insecurity and self-loathing like a new jacket—I zipped it up and tried to ignore the thick white body underneath. Every pound I gained, every drink I imbibed, every cup of chocolate chip cookie dough ice cream I swallowed with nausea and disgust. And then one day I tried a new strategy for weight loss.

If I couldn't lose weight through exercise, I would focus on diet. I began restricting and purging. My days belonged to the foods I did and did not eat: I did not eat breakfast. I did not eat snacks with lunch. I did eat a peanut butter and strawberry jelly sandwich every day for four years of high school. I did drink one eight-ounce bottle of water during school hours. I did eat a half a box of Oreo cookies.

I was often famished when I got home from school by 2:30 in the afternoon and would subsequently binge on some kind of sugary or salty snack. I'd eat as much as I could until I felt sick. And then, with the calories sitting in my belly like live grenades, I jammed my finger down my throat in the hope of setting them off. However, I could never make myself throw up. With the cold of the bathroom tile pressing into my knees, head bowed over the toilet as if in prayer, and pointer finger scraping the tear-shaped uvula at the back of my throat, I would sob. I sobbed at my failure to vomit, my failure to lose weight, my failure to fit into the size zero blue jeans that would qualify me as pretty.

But if I'm being honest, this poor body image did not begin as a teenager. Its insidious roots go back much further. I pulled a memory out of some deep place in the back of my mind as I wrote this book: I'm four-years-old standing in front of the full length mirror in my bedroom. I am wearing a blue and white leotard with white tights. I study my reflection. I see my profile and think that my body shape is too round. My belly looks like the semicircle I recently learned to identify. I am a half moon but half moons belong in the sky, not in little girl's bedrooms wearing leotards. I am four-years-old, and I don't like what my little girl body looks like in the mirror. My developing brain conjures the word chubby from somewhere. My vocabulary is limited, but I know this word. It is meant for stuffed animals and babies, but I am neither one of those things. My belly doesn't lay flat. It's supposed to be flat, I think. This memory makes me nauseous, not least of all because my own daughter is four, and I can't imagine her thinking she is anything but perfect when she looks at her body in the mirror.

It seemed that I would always need to lose "just five more pounds." I dropped weight when I went off to college. I had traded in the cardio I hated for the hot yoga I loved, but even with the new exercise, I still liked sugar at night—half a bag of Pepperidge Farm Sausalito cookies with my cup of Earl Grey tea as I binge-watched CSI Miami with my roommate. I liked pasta that was an easy and inexpensive dinner for a college girl living in her own apartment without the proximity of a dining hall. I liked pizza on Friday nights when my boyfriend came to visit. I also liked drinking too much and not running. "Carbs not cardio" would have been my mantra if I had one then.

When endometriosis arrived clutching my reproductive organs like a pearl necklace, hunger was disrupted. It was replaced with chronic bursts of pain that splintered my appetite into the crumbs I always wanted to subsist on but could never resist licking off my plate. At this point, I was in my twenties and had formed healthier workout routines and better eating habits. However, losing weight because of a chronic illness is certainly not the best way to lose weight and keep it off.

Because my history with my body is complicated and endometriosis was the lens through which I was forced to examine these body issues, it is, in essence, an unlikely liberator. Reevaluating my relationship with food and engaging in more meaningful choices that included organic, non-GMO, clean-eating and a gluten-free diet allowed me to finally eat in a satisfying way, maintain a healthy weight, and minimize endo pain. I had to relearn how to eat, how to enjoy drinking water, and finally bid adieu to late-night sugary snacks.

Reclaiming my body through my relationship with food was not as difficult as I thought it would be. When I decided to pursue alternative treatments to endometriosis, diet change was the very first action I implemented. Even before my appointment with the naturopath, I had begun to cleanse my palette and eliminate the sugar-laden foods, the genetically modified products, and the excessive carbohydrates that previously dominated my diet. Although I was a glutton for gluten and the thought of giving up everything—pasta, pizza, bagels—was not thrilling, I was committed to staying the course with these choices. I was also especially attached to dairy— daily yogurt, cheese on everything—so that restriction would also prove daunting. In practice, some gluten-free brands were a decent substitute for the fluffy, flakey breads I loved so much. Coconut milk yogurts were tasty, and oat milk was positively delicious (especially the extra creamy when you are craving something velvety divine). I also began avoiding red meat unless it was ground beef or a very high-quality, grass-fed cut. And, finally, incorporating more fruits and vegetables and paleo cuisine was simple and enjoyable. My endo pain was lessened and the change in diet also helped me maintain a healthy weight and feel more energetic overall. Endometriosis has had many roles in my life: arch-nemesis, stalker, Svengali and as it related to food, savior.

A few weeks into this new diet, a package arrived from my sister Jenny. Inside the box was a book *The Endometriosis Health & Diet Program*. Written by Dr. Andrew S. Cook and Danielle Cook, the holistic guide to managing endometriosis includes one hundred recipes. I also picked up several paleo cookbooks and found recipes online.

Dr. and Mrs. Cook seemed to substantiate my experience of going gluten-free and consuming primarily organic, Non-GMO foods writing in their book that "Pesticide exposure has been strongly associated with endometriosis; therefore, we recommend eating organic produce whenever possible." Additionally, the authors expound upon the inflammatory effect gluten has on the body and how that quality might trigger endo flare-ups. [20]

After reading their book, I came up with a manageable routine, a portrait of which looks like this: My morning begins with a hot bowl of steel-cut, gluten-free oatmeal. The sound of water simmering on the stove fills the quiet kitchen. The sunrise peeks in through the kitchen widow—pink and orange light stream in, teasing a beautiful day. The tea boiling in the kettle joins the morning chorus. I take my supplements—six tablets of Spirulina. I swallow the fishy-tasting pills without noticing their potent taste. I swig some warm water to wash them down.

The day unfolds in work or my daughter's activities depending on what day of the week it is. Around mid-morning, I eat a peanut butter breakfast bar. My little one notices that I'm eating something crunchy, and she asks for a bite. I gladly share. We both eat coconut milk yogurts a few minutes later—strawberry banana for her, raspberry for me. The thinner, less-creamy yogurt substitute is a little sweet and not as rich in flavor or consistency as regular yogurt, but it satisfies my dairy craving. If it is a teaching-day, I will inhale a breakfast bar and coconut milk yogurt in between classes or in my car right after class ends. I have recently started buying dairy-free fruit and veggie pouches—more smoothie than yogurt. They are so much easier to eat on the go, sans utensils. The brightly colored, anthropomorphized

---

20 Cook, Andrew S., and Danielle Cook. *The Endometriosis Health & Diet Program: Get Your Life Back*. Robert Rose Inc., 2017

carrots, apples, and strawberries are clearly meant for a younger consumer base, however, they are delicious regardless of age!

Lunch time rolls in around 1 pm. If I'm working, I'll likely grab a salad or quinoa bowl with grilled chicken. If I need a pick-me-up, I'll splurge on a kale smoothie or something similar. On days that I'm home, I attempt to make a dish similar to something I'd buy from a restaurant (but not the smoothie—there is way too much cleanup involved and they take too much time). I might also eat soup—lentil or veggie or, if it's cold and seasonal, a nice butternut squash soup. Gluten-free breads are really pretty tasty and can make for a nice sandwich if I'm feeling up for something more substantial. Toasting the bread creates a crispy, crunchy base which disguises the sandwich in such a way that it's almost like regular bread! Admittedly, I often add a slice or two of cheese to finish it off. A nice, hot cup of herbal tea pairs perfectly with lunch. Notes of raspberry from a raspberry leaf tea compliment most dishes.

3:30, 4 pm is the slump period. This time of day is defined by a dip in energy and, often, motivation. I inevitably need a boost at this point so I turn to a cup of matcha tea and nuts—pistachios or almonds—or a granola bar. If I need an extra salt-boost, I might turn to cauliflower crackers or gluten-free sweet potato tortilla chips.

I have my go-to meals that are easy and quick to prepare with minimal cleanup. My favorite, endo-friendly dinner dish is glazed salmon with rice and veggies. I make a gluten-free, soy-based glaze with honey and olive oil. Sometimes I add a little orange juice for a hint of citrus. The fish is seasoned with garlic powder and ginger. Throw it in the oven for twenty minutes or so, and, voila! I always double check rice brands to be sure they are gluten-free. Veggies like broccoli or carrots pair well with the main course. I keep them simple—broccoli gets some olive oil, garlic, salt, and pepper or carrots will be boiled with a tiny bit of butter and drizzled with maple syrup. This side dish is great if you are craving something a little sweet. The butter is a splurge but such a negligible amount never seems to bother me.

As the day winds down, the kitchen is cleaned up, my daughter is in bed, I'm cozy in yoga pants and a sweatshirt, on the couch, watching TV with my husband, I might indulge in a mug of extra creamy oat milk. It's thick and velvety, creamy like something forbidden—ice cream or a milkshake. Or if I'm craving something sweet, I'll nosh on some dark chocolate almonds which Greg inevitably steals, although I am happy to share them with him.

I am not rigid about following this diet. I am fastidious but I am human and sometimes a dairy craving can only be satisfied with a good, old fashioned vanilla milkshake. If there is one lesson I've learned from having endometriosis, it is to be gracious with myself. Living with chronic pain is difficult sometimes, but so too is living a holistic lifestyle. I might not feel like being healthy on a Saturday night when out to eat with my friends and everyone is indulging in verboten foods, and you know what? I just might join them. It is important to be understanding and forgiving with ourselves. We are human beings. Most of us haven't been eating or living this way before. It has taken years for this holistic lifestyle to become natural. And although I slip up from time to time, I've learned that a reckless eating or drinking day from time to time typically isn't that big of a deal. It is important to reward yourself, too. Life shouldn't be all pain and restriction; it should be delicious and delightful and positively satisfying.

10

DEPRESSION

According to a 2019 study by BBC and Endometriosis UK, 50% of women who suffer from endometriosis have had suicidal thoughts.[21] Living in chronic pain is more than simply being in constant, severe physical pain. It is not always having hope for relief. It is having no definitive cure. It is days that the pain is so bad you stay in bed and sob. It is deciding if you can handle simple, everyday tasks and then feeling joy when you can. It is depression. It is hopelessness. It it questioning whether you want to continue living with this pain—the

---

21 Xu, Juna. "50% Of Endometriosis Sufferers Have Suicidal Thoughts, New Study Finds." *Body and Soul*, 8 Oct. 2019, https://www.bodyandsoul.com.au/health/womens-health/50-of-endometriosis-sufferers-have-suicidal-thoughts-new-study-finds/news-story/ff57e5bfd7c88e60751ba2a136442af8

physical, the mental—this part of you that you never asked for or wanted. But it is also realizing that you can survive.

I was twelve-years old the first time I wanted to hurt myself. I imagined what it would feel like to take a pair of nail scissors to my wrists. It was a normal day; I'd just returned from the movies with a friend. I didn't understand why I felt so empty, so hopeless. I had two parents who loved me and two sisters I adored. I liked my small parochial school, and my friends had been in my life since we were in kindergarten. Despite the lack of setbacks and the almost fairy-tale quality of my life at this age, I was hurting. But I pretended I was fine and no one noticed anything amiss when I sat down at the kitchen table that night for dinner with my family. Mom made breaded pork chops and apple sauce. I cleaned my plate and chatted about school with my sisters before bed. They had no idea that earlier that afternoon I'd taken Mom's nail case out, found the pair of nail scissors, and traced the blue vein from the base of my hand down my wrist with the sharp point. I didn't push too deep, and I didn't actually draw blood. The only vestige of the incident was an ephemeral white line, a silhouette of an injury.

These feelings persisted throughout my teen years like a virus I just couldn't shake. I remember scenes from this time: I cried alone in my room. Linkin Park's *Hybrid Theory* played on a Discman. I listened to the songs on repeat through oversized headphones and ignored the rest of the world. I was a walking keep-out poster except no one knew I wanted them out. The days of quiet adolescent rebellions—secretly buying a thong from Victoria's Secret, sneaking into a club and dirty dancing with an older man whose name I never cared to learn—and the more serious mutinies: drinking inexpensive beer and whisky; lying to my parents about where I was and what I was doing; the disordered eating habits I hid from everyone.

Teenage angst is a common concept thrown around by frustrated parents and popularized by an English rock band from the mid '90s.

When hormones hijack a teenage brain and cause feelings of anxiety, fear, and rejection that mimic depression, teenage angst is typically the culprit. But these feelings of angst are more than existential. As a teenaged girl experiencing what I assumed was depression, I suffered from a potent sense of dread, and I hated myself because of these feelings. I endured these hormonal issues against a backdrop of loss and dysfunction. My grandmother, who was my closest friend and confidante, had passed away just before high school began. And then there was the slow-motion train wreck of my parents' marriage. These external factors certainly didn't help the internal cyclone of emotions and hormones.

Depression was not a word I ever used. Like endometriosis, it would be years before it became a part of my vocabulary, and when it did, it felt awkward and strange coming out of my mouth. This sadness was a part of me, an extra appendage. I tried to discard this word; I wanted to toss it into the trash like the tissues I used to dry the tears I pretended I wasn't crying. Depression. Chronic pain. These terms were not mine, I convinced myself. I pretended like they hadn't always belonged to me. But bouts of sadness, emptiness, pain—these things followed me around throughout my twenties, showing up with the vicissitudes of life: trauma, breakups, parent's divorce, professional limbo.

The emptiness inside me was an old friend I'd grown up with, but I had always done a very good job of keeping it a secret. I disguised pain with an outgoing personality and wore my smile like a weapon of defense. When chronic physical pain entered my life and tried to take over, I had more hurt to conceal from the outside world—so I did. I smiled often: at the woman who handed me my tea at the drive-thru Starbucks window; at the cashier in the grocery store; at the strangers I walked past in the hallway on my way to teach a class. I talked to everyone. And laughed. I always laughed. But sometimes on the inside, it was quiet and empty and echoed like a cave. It was murky too, like bats lived there. Sometimes, I thought that maybe they did. Maybe an entire colony of bats beat their wings and that's where the pain came from.

Pain pressed down hard like an anvil to my reproductive organs. It was as though I could feel every drop of blood, every cell, each rogue tissue and lesion festering on my ovaries and my bowel. Inflammation, irritation, scar tissue wrecked havoc and caused lower abdominal and pelvic pain. Sometimes, the pain squeezed all the happiness out of my life like it was orange juice and all that was left was an empty fruit shell. My life was a soft orange carcass and all the juice and sweet flesh had been discarded. Sex wasn't fun anymore because it hurt. Sleeping wasn't restful anymore because it hurt. Breathing wasn't desired anymore because it hurt. But then, relief would come.

My pain comes in many flavors: overwhelming, aggressive—shots of tequila in an empty stomach. Bitter, vomit-inducing, dizzying—cheap vodka straight from the bottle. Manageable but unpleasant and distracting—a mixed drink made with a cacophony of juices and too much sweet liquor.

I look into the mirror some days, and the eyes staring back at me are black holes where stars used to be. I wake up tired as if nighttime was made of flashing lights and loud music, and I spent it dancing. I'm tired all the time. I want to cry and sometimes I do but only in the car with the radio playing. Or at home when I'm alone. I've had heavy days before that sit on my chest until I'm about to suffocate. I've always had these gray days.

Once, a friend called me a girl of greens and grays. I liked this concept, this classification, and I embraced it, claimed it as my own, like a motto or coat of arms. Green like go—pain-free, no flare-ups of the physical or the mental pain. Green like freedom and happiness and pastoral dreams. And the gray—the color without any actual color, made up of black and white, the good and the bad, all the emotions and none of them. Gray—the overcast days, the days I just want to stay in bed and watch T.V.

And that is exactly who I am: I am a girl of greens and grays.

11

SEX & CHRONIC PAIN

What happens to your sex life when you suffer from chronic illness? The answer to this question is neither obvious nor simple. Nearly sixty percent of women with endometriosis experience pain during intercourse. This statistic, while shocking, is an unfortunate reality for many of us.[22]

Sometimes I experience only minor discomfort during sex—light cramping or an unpleasant tightening; other times the pain is so intense that it makes the act virtually impossible. Often the immense pleasure that comes with climax is immediately followed by equally

---

22 Elflein, John. "Endometriosis Impact on Sex Intimacy U.S. 2020." Statista, 10 Mar. 2022, https://www.statista.com/statistics/1241720/us-women-sex-intimacy-impacted-by-endometriosis/

immense pain in my abdomen and pelvic region. During these flare-ups, the only post-coital embrace I enjoy is with my pillow.

As I learned more about my endo-body, I began to understand that I could have very enjoyable, pain-free sex at certain times of the month. If I am fastidious with my holistic rituals, I can typically be healthy and comfortable enough for intercourse. However, when I do have flare-ups during sex, it's usually immediately following ovulation. In the days leading up to menstruation, I can almost always have pain-free sex. I've come to learn that my endometriosis seems to follow its own calendar, and I soon as I learned it's monthly routine, I was able to reclaim this part of myself again.

While I have been fortunate to get back to a normal, healthy sex life with only occasional endo interruptions, many other endo-warriors have been less lucky. For the purposes of this book, I looked into some additional ways that women can holistically reduce pain during intercourse. And this quest took me in a rather unexpected direction: pink frosted donuts.

Although I have yet to try the product, I discovered an online company called Ohnut which makes a wearable that customizes penetration depth and is specifically designed for women who experience pain during sex. The inventor apparently found inspiration by placing a frosted pink donut on a penis which led to immense physical relief during intercourse. According to their website, "Designed with renowned clinicians, Ohnut is a soft compressible buffer made from 4 rings, that can be used together or individually to adjust when penetration feels too deep, without sacrificing sensation."[23] The Ohnut is supposed to feel like skin, it is BPA, phthalate, and latex free, and made from FDA approved body-safe material.

In addition to maintaining holistic rituals to minimize occurrence of pain and products such as the Ohnut, there are a range of natural,

---

23 "How Ohnut Works." *OhnutCo*, https://ohnut.co/pages/how-it-works

essential oils and products that help alleviate pain during intercourse. These oil blends can include palm oil, coconut oil, evening primrose oil, and lavender oil among others. There are quite a few companies that make organic, natural products claiming to help with painful sex, but it is important to do your own research before using a new one (especially if you or your partner have any allergies). Greg is very allergic to coconut so anything that contains coconut oil could be a problem!

PELVIC FLOOR THERAPY

As defined by the International Society for Sexual Medicine, "Pelvic floor physical therapy is a treatment applied to pelvic floor muscles. Pelvic floor muscles support the pelvic organs, assist in bowel and bladder control, and contribute to sexual arousal and orgasm."[24] I had never heard of this therapy as an option for endometriosis sufferers until recently, but I was immediately fascinated. I learned that Pelvic Floor Therapy blends education with techniques such as pelvic floor exercises and biofeedback, manual therapy, electrical stimulation, and vaginal dilators. A natural, holistic approach to helping people improve muscle strength, improve flexibility, and learn about how their habits and hygiene could potentially be impacting sexual health. It is essentially physical therapy for the pelvic floor which is "s a group of ligaments, muscles, tendons, nerves and connective tissue that provides the base and support for the pelvic area. Additionally, "In women, the pelvic floor holds the bladder in the front, uterus at the top, and the vagina and rectum in the back." [25] It seems logical that

24 Betjes, Erik. "What Is Pelvic Floor Physical Therapy?" *ISSM*, 16 Dec. 2013, https://www.issm.info/sexual-health-qa/what-is-pelvic-floor-physical-therapy/

25 "Could Pelvic Floor Physical Therapy Help You? - Health & Wellness." *Loma Linda University Health*, https://lluh.org/patients-visitors/health-wellness/could-pelvic-floor-physical-therapy-help-you

this type of approach could potentially help someone suffering from chronic pain associated with endometriosis.

HORMONE-FREE BIRTH CONTROL APP

Although I used an app to determine ovulation so that I could try to get pregnant when my husband and decided it was the right time, Natural Cycles was a great method of birth control that offered 93% effectiveness and 98% effectiveness if used perfectly (that's the same as oral contraceptives!).[26] Not only do you learn about the unique characteristics of your cycle, this user -friendly app provides tailored insights and updates. Not only is it a great method of birth control, it is cleared by the FDA.

SEX, A COMPLICATED HISTORY

Attitudes towards sex evolve with knowledge, experience, age, and sometimes, chronic pain. I was raised Catholic. From the time I understood what sex was, probably around twelve-years-old, I also understood that well-behaved, moral girls didn't have sex until they got married. It was a sin, an act which would require confession, penance, forgiveness. However, I decided when I was still in high school that I was not going to wait that long; I would wait until I met someone I loved, someone who loved me.

I began to believe this endo pain was my punishment, my penance. My attitude towards sexual intercourse was casual and selfish for several years, and it was during this time that the pain began. I remembered reading Dante's Inferno as a college freshman. The concept of contrapasso—that hell is some perversion of the sin committed—seemed to take shape in my own life. The fifth Canto details The Second Circle of Hell where the lustful spend an eternity battered

---

26 "Natural Cycles Birth Control: No Hormones or Side Effects." *Natural Cycles*, 20 Oct. 2022, https://www.naturalcycles.com/

by violent storms. Dante writes, "...now here, now there, now down, now up, it drives them. There is no hope that ever comforts them—no hope for rest and none for lesser pain".[27] These ancient words so accurately captured the essence of my disease and the hopelessness that often went with it. When the endometriosis pain flared up, I felt as if pummeled by a violent internal storm. And for so many years, nothing comforted me, nothing lessened the pain. Was I lustful? My sin had been enjoyment of sex, therefore, my punishment was fitting: disruptive pelvic and abdominal pain, especially profound with climax. The residual Catholicism in my heart made me question: was endometriosis a Divine punishment? My contrapasso?

Sometimes in the throes of pain, I inhaled the agony, embraced it as my contrition. The Catholic doctrine in my brain searched for meaning in this experience. *This is corporeal penance, bodily mortification, a necessary result of my human imperfections,* I thought in the midst of a post-coital flare. *There is a direct relationship between the human body and the spirit, perhaps this pain will elevate me, let me access the deepest parts of my heart and mind. Attain God. Attain purification. This is penance. Forget ten hail Mary's or Our fathers. The Lord's prayer cannot bring me atonement the same way this corporeal penance can. The pain consumes me; my mind is sharp and clear like broken glass. It cuts to the soul and draws forgiveness.*

These thoughts preoccupied me from time to time, but, eventually, I let them go. I accepted that God was not punishing me with endometriosis. It was simply a disease that I, along with one in ten other women around the world, suffer from. But trying to find purpose in illness can be comforting. I am a woman who enjoys sex, and that's perfectly normal.

---

27 Alighieri, Dante, and Allen Mandelbaum. *The Divine Comedy of Dante Alighieri, Inferno: A Verse Translation, with an Introduction by Allen Mandelbaum.* Bantam Books, 1988.

12

FERTILITY & MOTHERHOOD

Fertility is a beautiful, complicated thing. As if sentencing women to a life of pain isn't enough, endometriosis also wrecks havoc on our reproductive organs, often compromising fertility. About 30-50% of women who have endometriosis suffer infertility.[28] In fact, the very little I understood of endometriosis before I was diagnosed with it was that it caused women to have difficulty conceiving. And because of these statistics, I was prepared to never become a mother.

---

28 Bulletti, Carlo, et al. "Endometriosis and Infertility." *Journal of Assisted Reproduction and Genetics*, Springer US, Aug. 2010, https://www.ncbi. nlm.nih.gov/pmc/articles/PMC2941592/#:~:text=Endometriosis%20 is%20a%20very%20common,endometriosis%20are%20infertile%20 %5B4%5D

Interestingly, the traditional Western treatment of endometriosis promotes solutions that essentially destroy a woman's fertility—at least temporarily. Birth control pills and Lupron injections—two options for managing this illness—halt the body's ability to get pregnant. The hormones in birth control pills stop ovulation and thicken the mucus on the cervix which prevents sperm from reaching an egg.[29] Lupron decreases estrogen production, stops ovulation and menstruation, and, essentially, mimics menopause. Besides surgery, these are the two most commonly proscribed treatments for endometriosis.

One can't help but wonder if it is the inherent misogyny present in Western medicine that dictates these methods of curbing fertility, treatments that should seem counterintuitive: stop a woman's body from reproducing, and it will fix her. How different is this, really, from lock her up in a room by herself to fix her hysteria, which, technically, can be anything ranging from difficulty sleeping to a fondness for writing. In the late 19th century, a Canadian psychiatrist went so far as to surgically remove a woman's uterus in order to "cure" her of mental illness.[30]

I spent a decade restricting my fertility. I shut it down with birth control pills in order to prevent unwanted pregnancy and reduce the length and discomfort of difficult periods. And it seems that it did keep my endo at bay for several years. But doesn't it, in a metaphysical sense, violate nature? How healthy can it actually be to trick your body into thinking it doesn't ovulate, that it can't have a baby? Isn't this,

29 Parenthood, Planned. "Birth Control Pills: The Pill: Contraceptive Pills." *Planned Parenthood*, https://www.plannedparenthood.org/learn/birth-control/birth-control-pill

30 Cohut, Maria. "Female Hysteria: The History of a Controversial 'Condition.'" *Medical News Today*, MediLexicon International, 13 Oct. 2020, https://www.medicalnewstoday.com/articles/the-controversy-of-female-hysteria#Vibrators-for-hysteria?

in a sense, gaslighting your body? The pills are after all manipulating normal, healthy functions.

During my quest for a diagnosis and effective treatment, I did encounter multiple doctors who touted pregnancy as a cure for endometriosis, which of course, leans into fertility instead of limiting it. However, when I was given this advice, my husband and I weren't ready to have a baby yet so it wasn't an option we considered—nor should it be considered as a treatment to a chronic condition. Babies shouldn't be conceived as a means to treat an illness. Babies aren't solutions to problems that need to be solved, and this is lazy medicine.

When I encountered Eastern medicine, I was struck by the emphasis on promoting fertility to treat endometriosis. This approach was the exact opposite of Western medicine. The herbal supplements, acupuncture, essential oils, teas, and even the diet seemed to make a woman more fertile—not less. The thinking was logical to me: a loving, nurturing approach always proved effective in other facets of life—friendship, teaching, dating—why not with chronic illness?

When I stopped taking birth control pills after being on them for nearly ten years, several things happened. My B-cup boobs shrank to an A-cup. Admittedly, this was a little disappointing (although I didn't mind the excuse to go bra shopping). My periods lengthened (from four days on the pill to almost seven). Cramping came back but was manageable with Midol and castor oil packs. And, perhaps most surprising of all, my libido increased dramatically—especially during ovulation.

Since the pill had been our primary method of contraception, my husband and I had to come up with a new form of birth control. We settled on a combination of the good, old fashioned pull out method plus figuring out when I was most fertile so we could be extra careful during those days, also known as the rhythm method. My Catholic grandparents would be so proud.

When Greg and I decided we were ready for a baby, I learned even more about my body. I downloaded an app to my phone that asked me questions every day about my period, general health, and temperature. It helped me track my periods and ovulation. This addition to my routine allowed me to delve deeper into understanding my endo experience than I had thought possible. It allowed me to document characteristics of my cycle, and, as it turns out, was helpful in documenting pain—like a kind of digital pain journal.

I learned of my body's natural cycle and the nuances, the subtle hints, the secrets she'd been whispering to me all along that I never bothered to listen to. These little details about the internal workings of my fertility were fascinating. As I tuned into the very specific timeline of my monthly cycle, I learned that my temperature rises slightly when I'm ovulating. I learned that when I experience endo pain, it will correspond with where exactly I am in my cycle (if I have pain, it will be worst the week after ovulation). I learned that I feel extra energetic and sexually-charged for the several days when I ovulate. I collected each bit of new information and used it to prepare myself for the next step: getting pregnant.

Before we officially started trying for a baby, I mentally prepared for the very real possibility that I would not be able to conceive naturally. I understood from the beginning of my endometriosis diagnosis that infertility is often a complication of the disease. I knew this, understood it, and accepted it. I decided that if a baby was meant to be, it would be. I had no interest in pursuing fertility treatments. I know many women who have gone down that road—some successfully and others not so successfully. These women are far braver and stronger than I will ever be. They are rock stars, goddesses, superhero women. I respect, admire, bow down to them. I can battle frequent pain, more than I thought I ever could, but I knew myself well enough to know that I could never withstand the mental strain, potential disappointments, the very real heartache of enduring injections, procedures, and possible negative pregnancy tests—or worse. I told Greg that I was unwilling to go down that road if it came to it, and like all of the complications of my disease that also impact him, he took it with grace.

I began trying the same way other non-chronically ill women do: I set out to determine when I was ovulating and got busy procreating! However, unlike healthy women, my process was threaded with equal parts doubt and additional holistic preparations. While most of my friends simply checked the calendar, tracked their periods, and poured a glass of wine to set the mood, I took my temperature each morning, took extra care to avoid inflammatory foods, and loaded up on Maca root—a supplement derived from a Peruvian vegetable and which, in my experience, boosted sex drive and fertility. It is important to note that Maca can stimulate estrogen production which may negatively impact endometriosis symptoms (although this did not appear to happen in my case).

And with shock, disbelief, and sheer joy, we learned that, after three months of trying, we were pregnant. While the pregnancy was not without its complications, the act of conceiving was not thwarted by endometriosis.

Pregnancy with endometriosis was challenging. I realized that I had become almost obsessive about my holistic regime and when I had to change it to accommodate the growing baby inside me, it caused me quite a bit of anxiety. All of a sudden the idea of healthy eating, gluten-free and low dairy intake was disgusting to me. I wanted carbs and dairy all the time, and I was not happy about it.

My belly was growing bigger by the day. My daughter was in breech position the entire time I was pregnant and we'd decided that I'd have a C-section. I noted the small, twin scars on either side of my abdomen from the laparoscopy I had several years earlier. I was prepared for a new addition to this collection of scars, the parts of my story that would be written in my skin, written with scalpels instead of ink. These marks would tell two stories of pain—one chronic and one singular, one that produced answers, one that produced a child. Both stories would grant answers to prayers—for medical validation and for a child of my own.

Pregnancy was difficult. By week four, I was nauseous all the time with frequent vomiting that occurred at all hours of the day, not just in the morning as its name suggested. The nausea finally dissipated at the end of the first trimester only to be replaced with exhaustion and severe anxiety. I was a hormonal mess, which probably contributed to the anxiety, but I'm sure that my sudden inability to adhere to my holistic regimen also contributed. Before pregnancy, I drank my herbal teas, took supplements and followed a precise, clean, gluten-free diet. I exercised regularly and had acupuncture appointments. During pregnancy, I couldn't drink all the teas I was used to, had to stop the supplements because my doctor recommended it, and suddenly only wanted to eat foods that were off-limits. I also stopped acupuncture and couldn't motivate myself to workout after week sixteen. The thought of a salad or gluten-free, dairy-free meal was suddenly revolting. I craved macaroni and cheese like my body craved oxygen. I would have lived off it if I could. But even though I'd strayed from my holistic rituals during pregnancy, I had stopped having flare-ups. Perhaps the doctors were correct—pregnancy could ultimately alleviate endometriosis.

I remember the morning in early October very clearly: I was twenty-nine weeks pregnant and teaching a freshmen composition class at a Jesuit university in Connecticut. During the class, I began experiencing sharp, cramping pain—similar in some respects to the endo pain I was accustomed to but hadn't experienced since conceiving my daughter in March. This pain continued throughout class and afterwards. I was supposed to drive to the second college where I taught in the afternoon, but I thought I should check in with my gynecologist first. The nurse I spoke with over the phone thought it would be a good idea to come in just to err on the side of caution.

As I sat in my doctor's office in the middle of a bright autumn afternoon, hooked up to a machine that measured the strength of my contractions, I panicked. These contractions were very close together and consistent in length and strength. I was sent to the hospital where Greg eventually joined me. My daughter wasn't born that day, but I was put on bed rest and continued contracting for the next seven weeks. In addition to endometriosis, I also have hyperthyroid condition, specifically Grave's Disease. These comorbid conditions made me a high risk pregnancy despite only being in my early thirties.

I spent the last seven weeks of pregnancy uncomfortable and generally frustrated and anxious. It didn't help that Greg was in the hospital with kidney stones (twice!) during this time and we were selling our house. The nursery wasn't set up, I was forced to work remotely and drop most of the classes I had been teaching, and mostly, I was scared shitless.

The doctor sliced into my abdomen during a C-section in the early morning hours of a cold November day. The minute my girl was pulled from my body, I felt like I could breathe. My body was mine again. After seven weeks of contractions, bed rest, and the sudden burst of water in the middle of the night at thirty-six weeks pregnant, my baby was born. Although groggy with drugs and hormones and emotions, I remember the doctor coming into the recovery room not long after the delivery to tell me that she did not see any evidence of endometriosis while performing the cesarean-section to deliver my daughter. While feeling relieved at this news, in that moment, I hardly considered it important. My mind was focused on this beautiful, tiny, five-pound human that my body had brought into the world. In spite of suffering from an illness that leaves many women battling infertility, I created life. I was in awe.

In the early morning hours, my daughter wakes. I prepare her bottle, cradle her in my arms and feed her. As she touches my lips with one chubby hand, the other holds onto her white muslin blanket with the lion print—her blankie. I try to smile and interact with her like I normally do. *How was your sleep, baby girl? What do you want to do today?* However, this particular morning I am in agony, in the middle of a flare-up, and all I can do is watch the formula slowly leave the bottle and pray she drinks faster. In this moment, all I want to do is grab my heating pad and go into the bathroom. These precious, short-lived 6 a.m. moments that I cherish so much were wasted this morning; I spent them distracted and focused on breathing through the pain radiating in my abdomen. In this moment, I felt like an awful mother.

Endometriosis pain is bad, but when exacerbated by guilt—it is unbearable. Working mothers often talk about the guilt they feel not being around for every day events—big or small, something I'm familiar with as well. But it's an altogether different brand of guilt when you are present but still absent. Although it may not be selfish, it is still devastating.

When I stopped breast feeding at about seven weeks and I had yet to experience an endometriosis flare-up, I thought I was in the clear. However, at exactly three months post-partum, the endometriosis came back with a vengeance. I had been asleep in the short, intervening hours between late-night feedings. While the sleep was light, the kind of disrupted, nervous slumber that belongs to new parents, I woke with a start. It took me a full minute to realize that the baby was still fast asleep, her tiny fist above her head, free from the tight swaddle my husband and I had practiced even before her birth. She was not crying; I was startled awake by a familiar pulsing, radiating pain in my abdomen.

Of course new motherhood is busy; there is no time for the things you had so much time for before such as siting down and enjoying a hot cup of tea while you read the morning headlines. Now, I make a cup of tea and it's ice cold before I finish it two hours later. It's still possible to eat healthy and gluten-free, and once I stopped breast-feeding, I was able to resume my herb and tea regimen. I'm slowly easing back into my holistic rituals and lifestyle focused on Eastern medicine; however, there are still some days that I experience pain that takes my breath away. I'll be reading to my little one, and it will come on, unexpectedly and all at once. I'll put the baby down in her pack n' play and rush off to the bathroom. Sometimes relieving my bladder helps with the pain's intensity. New mothers are expected to be tired, but not from sleep interrupted by episodic pain. The time you have to sleep as a new parent is precious so spending it awake, curled up with a heating pad, and reading Facebook headlines is not ideal.

When I look into my daughter's eyes, I think about all the things I want to protect her from. One of those things is endometriosis. As I care for her through my own pain, I pray that she never has to experience this suffering. I pray that it isn't genetic. *Let her inherit my sense of humor. My love of reading. Please, let her never experience chronic pain.*

Things have slowly returned back to normal, or, that is, to a new normal. Life before my daughter is very different from life with her. My relationship with my body and my pain is different too. I have a new scar to go along with the small, white twin lines decorating my lower abdomen. I look at these scars in the mirror and read them like lines in a story—a story about a woman's pain *and* joy. The joy of motherhood. These scars are also gratitude and perseverance and defiance. I challenged my body to create life in spite of a condition that could and often does complicate this ability. Pain sneaks into my days and tries to dominate them but fails. Again and again I will get through it; I will control it with my alternative methods; I will ignore it, and I will concentrate on my daughter and the way she moves her tiny hands when she wants something, the way she smiles at me when I sing to her in my off-key voice. My endo exists and will likely continue to live in the organs inside me. But it isn't who I am, it doesn't define me as a woman or as a mother. My daughter is my world, and, with or without endometrioses, she is ultimately all that really matters.

13

NOT YOUR AVERAGE PAINSOMNIA

The house at two a.m. is quiet. The only sounds are the soft snoring of my daughter on the baby monitor and the old dog's heavy breathing from his bed in our room. My husband appears to be sleeping peacefully beside the spot where I usually lay curled up and tangled with him. I've only been out of bed for a minute, but he's already replaced me with a pillow—hugging the fluffy ersatz wife in a way that makes me envious.

The pain woke me like a grenade—sudden, violent, and catastrophic. It erupted in the lower, left-side of my abdomen. I transitioned from sound asleep to wide awake in a matter of seconds. It is June 2021. It has been five years since I first learned I had endometriosis. Since a doctor first sliced into me. I live most days pain-free, but there still are occasional flare-ups that hit me like a drunk driver collision. Most often, these episodes occur in the middle of the night.

Please not this. Not again. I silently beg my body, but, as expected, it ignores me as I make my way to the bathroom. I know what's coming. I'm prepared for it—mentally and physically. This is a battle I've fought before. I gather my weapons: heating pad, cell phone, and space. The cold tile of the bathroom floor waits for me to take my position. I kneel down, tuck my knees into my chest, plug the pad in and place it under my shirt on the bare skin. *Burn away pain.* I take out my cell phone. It's 2:34 am. *Let's rock and roll* I think, smiling briefly at my daughter's newest favorite phrase and its current relevance.

But this night is not ordinary, not the average nighttime painsomnia. It begins as familiar—the stabbing, throbbing, cramping in the lower left-side by the ovary. The initial build-up of the painful sensation is normal at first, but after a few minutes, it takes an unexpected and dramatic turn: it continues escalating. It amplifies to the point where my entire body is cold and sweating. I vomit from the intensity of the pain. I am so overwhelmed with pain and sweat and chills and vomiting that I tear my nightshirt off—this is the only action I can take. I am helpless but removing my clothes is doing something and I need to do something. I am naked and crying in supplication on the bathroom floor; as if in prayer, a martyr begging God to ease this pain. I cannot take any more. I pray for death. I pray for an ending. I pray for anything but this pain.

I am down on all fours, grunting and whining like an animal. The pain has reduced me to this primal position, whimpering like road kill in the last seconds of its life. This is what endometriosis has reduced me to—I am less than human. I am the manifestation of pain itself; They say endo is the worst pain a woman can experience outside of cancer. This is greater than seven weeks of contractions, a C-section, and a laparoscopy all rolled into one. The pain is destructive—it feels as though my rectum is ripping in half. I remember that my doctor had told me once, years ago, that she removed endo lesions from my bowel. This must be them; they must have come back. This is their comeback, the Revenge of the Bowel Lesions (not quite as catchy, as say, Revenge of the Sith) but if the Sith from Star Wars were to invade a human body—this is what it would feel like. The Sith—a dark, insidious, antagonist in a science fiction world seems like a fitting metaphor. With their red skin—red like human blood, and the bone spurs that decorate their faces, these beings are the epitome of evil, an endometriosis lesion personified. I wonder if serenity and detachment can conquer it—let me become a Jedi.

After some time (it is hard to keep track of how much passes when in this kind of pain-induced fever dream), my husband knocks on the door. It has been many months since I've risen in the middle of the night, since I experienced this symptom of endometriosis: the painsominia.

He is more than worried: I can hear the fear in his voice. I haven't heard this distinct note of terror since I went into pre-term labor with our daughter two and half years earlier. I can hardly articulate a response when he asks, "What's wrong?" I mostly grunt and sob, I'm inchoate, an animal wounded and primal. This pain is primal. I'm nothing more than a body with flesh and organs and they are dying inside me, they must be dying inside me. But when he adds, "Let's take you to the hospital." I manage a more articulate response: clear, definitive, angry I spit out, "No."

I refuse to go to the emergency room again. I know how the montage will play out: I will sit, in pain and shaking, ignored by the flustered receptionist and overworked nurses. The other patients surrounding me will be irritated and impatient. Eventually, I'll be seen by a nurse who will ask the standard litany of questions regarding medical history and current symptoms. They'll leave me and my pain in the room alone again and cold, the air in the hospital is always dry and arctic. There will be more waiting. A doctor will see me. They will suggest tests to eliminate anything too serious—likely an intravaginal ultrasound—and then I'll be told to take some over the counter medications to manage the pain. The entire thing will play out while the pain isn't helped at all and then I'll be billed some obscene amount despite the fact that I have insurance.

"Are you sure? Something is really wrong," Greg insists, desperate to help but helpless just the same.

"Yes." I can only manage a monosyllabic response, but I'm insistent.

"What can I do?" The love and concern in his voice almost breaks my heart—if my heart hadn't been pounding so hard and already breaking from my body's betrayal.

"Nothing. Please leave me alone." I feel like I'm being harsh, but I can't manage sweet or grateful while I'm lying on the bathroom floor, drenched, shaking, in pain, and praying for an end.

It is in these pain-filled moments that the toll of chronic pain can be seen on the faces of loved ones. I'm not the only one in pain—my husband is too. This pain is different from mine, of course, but it is real and it is devastating. Helpless to alleviate the pain of a suffering loved one is an altogether different but still potent chronic condition.

"I'm so sorry, Sweetie," he says, voice made of cracking glass not yet shattered. He retreats to the bedroom where I know he won't be able to go back to sleep.

The pain reaches a climax. It is too much for my body to handle and I vomit again. Acid burns my throat; tears leak from my eyes. I am naked, skin slick with sweat, hands hardly able to hold onto the side of the toilet bowl as I evacuate my stomach. I concentrate on my breathing. I try to remember yoga and the emphasis on inhale, exhale, deliberate and powerful breath. Breath can center you. Heal you. Empower you. At least that's what I vaguely recall in the middle of the night, mid pain-attack after nearly a decade since practicing yoga.

Eventually, the pain subsides. About a half hour has passed since I was woken from sleep. The fist around my insides loosens its clutch.

I'm cold without my clothes on so I get myself dressed again. As I climb back into bed beside my now awake husband, I begin shaking—more than a tremble or chills. It's that quake, that uncontrollable, full body shudder that happens after a body experiences a trauma—like childbirth. It passes after a minute or two and the tension in my muscles dissipates. It's over. For now.

In the morning, I feel like myself again. I wake, take my vitamins, drink a hot cup of matcha green tea and eat a small bowl of gluten-free, steel cut oatmeal with a drizzle of maple syrup. I notice the cumulous clouds smudging the sky and listen to my daughter laugh at her morning cartoons. The dog begs for food at my feet. This is a beautiful, normal pain-free morning—no evidence of the previous night's trauma can be seen anywhere except perhaps in the slight puffiness in my eyes.

I'm filled with post-traumatic reflection: this wasn't an average episode of painsomnia. I am intimate with the nuances of my condition, each note of pain—cramp, sharp, piercing jab, radiating and mild or barbaric, Inquisition-level torture of my pelvic area—I have memorized these feelings like the lyrics of a favorite song. I know which foods trigger episodes of endometriosis. I know how stress impacts these flares. I also know how a rupturing ovarian cyst feels—the momentum. This kind of pain comes on just as suddenly as endo but it crashes, overtakes my body faster and harder and longer, a tsunami of pain destroying anything in its wake. This pain is catastrophic, nonstop gut-punches on methamphetamine. Endo pain is enduring, drawn out, more consistent cycles. Cysts are similar but more overwhelming, debilitating with a more definitive ending. Although they can return, typically, once a cyst has ruptured the pain leaves your body. I realize that last night's episode was more similar to a rupturing cyst (the climax of my endo pain is never quite that severe, and I typically don't throw up from it). However, because the pain was unusually bad, I decide I should play it safe and see a doctor.

I had decided to visit my regular gynecologist after this incident. It felt serious in a way that made me nervous. It was more severe, felt more destructive than my normal pain. It felt prudent to visit a gynecologist instead of a naturopath.

At the time, I was seeking a local naturopath as the commute to Massachusetts had become nearly impossible as a working mom. Yes, I was a convert to the holistic lifestyle, however, I never dismissed Western medicine entirely. I also suffer from hyperthyroidism and successfully manage it with good old-fashioned drugs prescribed by an endocrinologist I happened to really like. While the laparoscopy ultimately failed to help my endo pain, I can't ignore the fact that I had the procedure a few months before beginning a holistic regime. It is certainly possible that my Eastern methods wouldn't have been as successful without the lap. And perhaps most of all, I am a typical American woman—a patient of Western doctors for my entire thirty-five years of life, raised on the belief that doctors are who you see when you are sick or hurting. This ideology isn't so easily erased.

And so, although this relationship with Western medicine has often bordered on abusive—neglectful, dismissive, cruel, and, at times, rendering decisions and tests that ultimately hurt me—I went back. Maybe they won't be so awful to me this time. Maybe they really do love me.

I scheduled an appointment with my gynecologist for the next afternoon. The doctor was a handsome, middle-aged man with salt and pepper hair. Laugh lines framed his rich, maple syrup eyes but they did not smile at me that afternoon. Although the bottom of his face was obstructed by his black mask, I imagined a thin, unsmiling mouth behind it. He entered the room, gave a rushed polite greeting, and got down to business. I told him of my experience, the pain, the duration, the intensity. I briefly mentioned my history with endometriosis and cysts and suggested that it was probably a cyst, but I wanted to make sure there was nothing else potentially serious going on.

He bristled at the mention of what I believed had happened, annoyed that I had the audacity to play doctor. I was sure he'd experienced his fair share of Internet doctors—WebMD devotees who perhaps dishonored his profession by googling their symptoms and diagnosing themselves. Of course, this is not at all what I was doing. It was after all, my body, my history, my pain. I know it better than anyone else. Didn't he want to take advantage of my insider knowledge?

While I was annoyed at his annoyance, I was most upset by what came next. After completing a quick pelvic exam, he decided that I was obviously fine and no further testing was needed. He said, "The next time you experience pain like that, just take some Aleve or over-the- counter medication, and that should help. You'll be fine." As if I hadn't thought to take Aleve myself. As if this pain was just a silly headache, and I just needed to sleep it off. As if I was just some silly girl with silly pain who had wasted ten minutes of his very important, valuable time. Silly me. I should have known better. Why had I expected different? Why hadn't I learned my lesson?

The follow-up with the gynecologist left me with a seventy-six-dollar balance after insurance and festering resentment. I know my body like a favorite song played on repeat. Every lyric and note, the feelings it invokes—familiar. If something is out of tune, I know it. I know that this was a cyst that ruptured. I know this because I know the difference between the regular, consistent humming of endo pain and the cataclysmic throbbing of a rupturing cyst. In my gut, I already diagnosed this event, but I wanted acknowledgement, confirmation from a medical professional, reassurance of this diagnosis and that it was over for now. Pain is traumatic but so too is consistent dismissal of your pain by doctors, by the people we have been taught to turn to when we are sick. But then, history has shown us that doctors have mistreated women for centuries. This is nothing new. This is just as much a tradition in Western medicine as the practice of healing.

I left the doctor's office angry that I had wasted my time, scolded myself for thinking it would be different, and determined that I was done this time. Enough is enough.

14

ENDOMETRIOSIS: A FAMILY AFFAIR

We weave stories from aunts and cousins to create a quilted narrative, a family history that reveals mysterious pain, infertility, and painful periods. These are not the bedtime stories we tell our children or the ones we exchange around the tree at Christmas time, but they are equally important, if not vital to our genealogy. These are shared in hushed tones and whispers, as if it is not appropriate to tell them at all, as if they are more dirty secrets than stories of our inheritance.

My sister Jenny was the first person who suggested there might be another way to treat endometriosis. She gave me hope when Western Medicine had shattered it. Jenny embodied the holistic lifestyle she touted as an alternative for my pain, and so, it was especially devastating when our roles seemed to switch.

In Fall 2021, a late afternoon phone call with my sister began just as another conversation: what's new? How's mom? Have you talked to Dad? And the litany of quotidian catching-up. Then an unexpected twist: How did you know when you had endometriosis? And next: a pit in my stomach.

Jenny told me of a recent incident where she was a guest at a wedding, and she had enjoyed a rather gluttonous amount of delicious steak tips. That night and into the next morning, she was plagued with horrible pain in her abdominal and pelvic area. She used a heating pad, took some Aleve, and rested a bit before it eventually passed and she was able to head into work. What did I think this was? A cyst maybe?

It broke my heart that my little sister was experiencing debilitating pain that was so similar to the kind I'd become intimately familiar with. She later explained that although she'd recently had a routine visit with her gynecologist, she did not feel comfortable bringing this issue up to her. She added, "it seemed like she was busy, distracted. I didn't want to bother her. It didn't seem important."

How often do we do this? How often do we not feel comfortable to discuss our true, unfiltered health issues with a medical professional? I'd long suspected that my younger sister also suffered from endometriosis. For years, she'd complained of extremely painful, almost debilitating periods and the latest flare-up triggered by the consumption of red meat confirmed it in my mind. I had mentioned years earlier that she should ask her gynecologist about endometriosis. Back then, she'd taken my advice and raised the possibility with the gynecologist she was seeing at that time. Jenny said upon completion of her routine pelvic exam, the doctor stated that she didn't detect any evidence of endo. My sister had no idea a doctor can't diagnose endo with a simple pelvic exam and that, in fact, the only definitive way to diagnose is with surgery. This of course suggested that the doctor was either an idiot, lazy, or just indifferent. There was no uncertainty, however, as to what I was upon hearing about her experience: enraged.

It was my turn to be the frustrated and helpless loved one of a chronic pain sufferer, but with an exception: I had tools that others don't have: I have years of my own experience with alternative treatments and a plethora of knowledge gleaned from research, online support groups, and many conversations with fellow endo warriors. Jenny wasn't alone and she didn't need to suffer the same indignities that I (and most women with chronic illness) do at the hands of Western medicine.

It felt good being able to listen to my sister and her pain narrative. I felt like I was helpful in suggesting teas to try and herbs that I've found alleviate the pain. She already lives a healthy lifestyle including eating a paleo diet (gluten and dairy-free), a reason I believe she's been able to keep her endo relatively in check for so many years.

Although research into family incidence of endometriosis is ongoing, an article published in 2020 by *Medical News Today* suggest that it can affect women in the same family—potentially. "A 2010 study included 80 participants with endometriosis and 60 without it. Those with endometriosis were more likely to have a relative with the condition. About 5.9% of participants with endometriosis had a first-degree relative with the condition, compared with just 3% of those without the health issue. While the likelihood of having a relative with the condition was almost doubled in the endometriosis group, the likelihood was still very low." The article highlights the history of lack of information and understanding by the medical community when it comes to endometriosis writing that "many doctors were ill-informed about endometriosis until recently, and it often went misdiagnosed. Some research indicates that as many as 70% of cases in the 1970s were undetected. This means that mothers and other relatives of people with endometriosis may have had the condition but never received a diagnosis." [31]

Even though this article was written in 2020, the study was done in 2010, included only eighty participants, and appears to be the most recent one done on the topic. Lack of research coupled with lack of diagnoses correlates to very little information regarding the occurrence of endometrioses among family members. Although I have no scientific evidence to substantiate the experiences of multiple family members, I have curated anecdotal evidence that suggests the likelihood of endometriosis within my immediate family.

Kristina is my first cousin on my mother's side. She grew up far from me—on naval bases in Japan and other parts of the world before settling in Maryland. I remember overhearing mom and grandma discussing how she was often sick and had a brutal monthly visitor, but I was young and didn't really understand what this meant. Kristina would later candidly share the details of her gruesome experience with endometriosis, one that has included heavy, painful periods, bloating, and, eventually, a hysterectomy that did not resolve her endo pain.

My forty-six-year-old cousin was diagnosed with endometriosis in 2006 via exploratory laparoscopic surgery at the age of thirty-one. Prior to surgery, she experienced painful, irregular periods with clotting. She had two more surgeries before deciding to have a complete hysterectomy in 2013. Even after having her uterus removed, she still endured pain five years later. Another surgery was then performed and determined that there was still evidence of some endometriosis as well as massive scar tissue on some of her organs. Although her endometriosis was described as "moderate," her years

---

31 Villines, Zawn. "Is Endometriosis Hereditary? Research and Statistics." *Medical News Today*, MediLexicon International, 12 Feb. 2020, https://www.medicalnewstoday.com/articles/is-endometriosis-hereditary #is-it-hereditary

of suffering were marked by unbearable pain that often led to trips
to the emergency room.

My maternal grandmother became easily pregnant with two babies
after she married my grandfather in 1950. But when they tried for a
third, nothing happened. After years of trying without luck, Grandma
Mary made peace with the fact that she wouldn't have the big family
she'd wanted. She didn't ask questions and accepted it as God's plan
for her. Eventually, she did give birth to a third child. He arrived
twelve years after my mother, when she and her brother were heading
into their teen years. Although endometriosis was never brought
up by my grandma nor was she one to share the intimate details of
menstruation, she was, after all, a good Irish Catholic girl who would
never talk about such things, I cannot help but wonder if she too,
suffered from endometriosis. There is, of course, no way to know this,
and it is purely speculation. If my grandmother were still alive today,
I'm not sure she'd be willing to discuss these personal medical topics.
She was a nurse and certainly comfortable with bodies, blood, illness,
and medicine; however, Grandma Mary was raised Catholic during a
time that did not allow for open conversations about sex and sexual
health. I imagine if I'd ever asked her about her period, she'd likely
have laughed and dismissed the question with a "now why on earth
would you need to talk about that!"

If we were to go back in time, retrace the histories of our female
ancestors, what kind of stories would we learn? Would they talk of
chronic pain and heavy periods and difficulty conceiving? I will never
know of course, because these are not the kinds of stories families
share around the dinner table. It is not the sort of family narratives
that have ever mattered. That is, until now.

15

ENDOMETRIOSIS IN THE ERA OF COVID-19

We live in an age of misinformation, disinformation, constant debate and disagreement. It is a time marred by fear, ignorance, doubt and general social malaise. I don't think it is possible to write this book in the age of COVID-19 without addressing how this disease and the vaccine factor into the endometriosis and chronic illness dialogue.

The impact of the virus and the vaccine on women suffering from endo has raised many questions. Some women began complaining of changed periods after receiving the vaccine including post-menopausal women. Other women complained of complications and elevated levels of endometriosis pain. Some endo-warriors had similar complaints after suffering from the virus itself—unrelated to the vaccine. Only one thing seemed certain early on in the pandemic: menstruation and women's health has often been overlooked in medical discussions and studies. However, in 2021, we finally had a moment when our voices were heard: the FDA announced that it would devote millions of dollars to research the vaccine's impact on menstruation. Not an insignificant victory indeed!

The hot topic of discussion in online support groups seemed to be universal: has the vaccine effected your endometriosis? From what I read and learned, some women have suffered a dramatic increase in endo-flares and pain. One woman wrote, "It was the worst endo pain I'd ever experienced. I ended up in the Emergency Room." Although some women discussed seeing worsening symptoms, others saw had no discernable impact whatsoever. This information was gleaned primarily from reading articles and following conversations in several online support groups for endo-sufferers. Almost all the women who had experienced some menstrual changes or flare-ups noted that this was temporary—typically around three to four months.

In August 2021, Michigan State University announced that it would be studying the potential effects of both the virus and the vaccine on menstruation. An article from *MSU Today* states,

> Researchers led by a Michigan State University professor will conduct two studies of whether infection with the COVID-19 virus or vaccination to prevent COVID-19 is affecting the menstrual cycles of women and girls. The studies, funded by the National Institutes of Health, follow anecdotal reports by some women that they had heavier or irregular menstrual cycles after they were infected with the virus or inoculated against it.[32]

32 Kelley, Geri. "Researchers to Study Possible Link between COVID-19 and Menstrual Changes." *MSU Today*, 30 Aug. 2021, https://msutoday.msu.edu/news/2021/researchers-to-study-possible-link-between-covid-19-and-menstrual-changes

These initial reports provided evidence echoed by much of my own anecdotal research. It is reassuring that studies are underway to learn what, if any, changes are occurring to periods from COVID and the vaccine. The study will examine if either contributes to heavier or irregular periods and/or pelvic pain.

Another study was published in March 2022 that had more concrete data. A cross-sectional investigation of menstrual symptoms after COVID19 vaccine performed by Jordan University Hospital in Amman, Jordan found that about 66% of the participants in the study reported menstrual symptoms after the first dose of the vaccine. The conclusion of the study was that there is a possible link between the COVID-19 vaccine and menstrual abnormalities that have impacted quality of life.[33] However, it was also found that in about 93% of these women the symptoms resolved within a two month period.

While most of the anecdotal evidence and even the study focused on women ranging in age from early twenties to mid forties, these abnormalities also appear to effect postmenopausal women. I personally know a woman in her mid-sixties who experienced severe cramping, bloating, and breakthrough bleeding after receiving her vaccine. She described the symptoms as "like getting her period again after more than a decade." It was uncomfortable, strange, and very unsettling. However, these abnormalities only lasted about two months. Upon further investigation, I came across multiple articles in various international publications which described similar symptoms in postmenopausal women after receiving the COVID-19 vaccination. In all incidents, the changes and symptoms dissipated within a few months.

---

33 Muhaidat, Nadia, et al. "Menstrual Abnormalities after COVID-19 Vaccine: IJWH." *International Journal of Women's Health*, Dove Press, 28 Mar. 2022, https://www.dovepress.com/menstrual-symptoms-after-covid-19-vaccine-a-cross-sectional-investigat-peer-reviewed-fulltext-article-IJWH

I contracted COVID-19 before I received the vaccine. After I had recovered from the virus, the first significant change I noticed regarding menstruation was that I did not ovulate for a month. This was followed by a month of what felt like "extra ovulating"—prolonged and extreme heavy ovulation symptoms such which lasted for up to six days. I also experienced a slight spike in endo pain after COVID infection. This uptick in pain was still manageable especially compared to some of the other long haul symptoms like hair loss and altered taste and smell. My period also became heavier and lasted longer. These menstrual changes only lasted a couple months and were relatively minor.

I waited about five months after the infection before receiving the vaccine. Upon getting the jab, I experienced an increase in frequency and severity of endometriosis pain. However, the worst symptom was the change to my period which became heavier, longer, and very irregular. This menstrual change lasted about four months. Admittedly, it was very frustrating, but I was able to manage the setback by focusing on the fact that most of the anecdotal evidence I'd found indicated this shift would be temporary. And, thankfully, it was. That is, until I became infected with COVID-19 a second time.

My second round with the virus was not as severe as the first time around, however, the period changes that occurred post-virus were as bad as after the vaccine and they lasted just as long. Another four months of extremely heavy bleeding, bloating, and cramping followed recovery from COVID. Again, enduring these menstrual irregularities was frustrating but bearable—especially given the other long-term symptoms that I could have experienced and, thankfully, didn't.

Ultimately, based on my research and personal experience, both COVID-19 and the vaccine seem to impact menstruation and endometriosis, but only temporarily. The pandemic exposed some brutal truths and inequities in the medical industry; however, the disturbing lack of attention and concern for the varying ways a virus or vaccine could impact menstruation and women's health issues has been brought to light. And the optimist in me believes this will bring about important and necessary change. One silver lining in an otherwise dark period.

16

DIGITAL KINSHIP

I've never really believed in therapy. Perhaps it's because it didn't work for my parents when they tried marriage counselling a year or so before their divorce. Perhaps it's because when my parents made my sisters and me see this same counselor, the only feeling I left with was irritation that I had wasted an hour of my time. Perhaps it is because I've always been lucky to have a coterie of women in my life, an inner circle of friends who listened and gave appropriate advice when life dealt unexpected or unfortunate blows. They helped me weather broken hearts, my parents' divorce, and the typical stress of being a young woman—that is, until they couldn't.

When I was suffering from undiagnosed pain in my twenties, it wasn't something any of my girlfriends had experienced. They couldn't understand the kind of visceral agony I experienced on a regular basis or the corresponding emotional suffering. This wasn't familiar territory to any of us. No one talked about chronic pain then, and no one knew I was going through this kind of illness and severe pain.

When I was a young girl, the only mention of endometriosis was in passing or overheard. My mother once talked about her best friend's difficulty conceiving a baby. She mumbled something about a condition that had caused her friend's struggle. There were also the occasional conversations between adult women about "girl problems" that would find their way to listening little ears. These vague references to a serious illness were all I heard of endometriosis. The snippets of eavesdropped conversations and ambiguous references taught me that people weren't comfortable talking about this illness. Forget about Bruno—it's Endo we don't talk about.

Endometriosis. When the doctor first uttered this word, I thought it sounded like a sexually transmitted disease or some kind of foreign bacteria or maybe a plant. The word itself was frightening and mysterious; the lack of knowledge I had about it reinforced that notion. It was fear, darkness, isolation. This word lodged in my throat until I choked on it. I was alone. Whoever had heard of such a thing?

But this is 2022. The age of Me Too and reckonings and Trump, but also Ruth Bader Ginsberg and Michelle Obama and Oprah. We rise. We fight. We find each other and share our stories and the lessons we've learned from our experiences. What treatments work. What doesn't. More then that, we listen and understand each other when no one else can or will.

I found companionship online. Facebook, a place notorious for harboring misinformation and internet trolls, offered me a community of women I didn't even know I needed. I participated. I learned and shared and we educated each other when society didn't. We became more than simply a support group or network of women exchanging tips and information. We understood each other when our closest friends or relatives didn't. We provided the advice our doctors failed to give us. In one group, I read about women who didn't experience relief after laparoscopies or hysterectomies. In another thread, a woman talked about the holistic herbs and essential oils she found helpful in managing her pain. A kind of digital kinship sprang up from shared pain, grew through the cracks left by Western Medicine and ineffective treatments. The nexus was suffering but what blossomed was support and even friendship.

This is the new sisterhood I became a part of. I wrote a column for an online publication, published essays on my story and quest for holistic healing. Women who read about my experience began reaching out via email. Some shared their stories, some asked questions and sought advice, and some simply thanked me for sharing my story. This surprising outreach was unexpectedly comforting. My illness didn't simply belong to me anymore—it belonged to every person who read these publications.

As with most things related to the internet, there is a dark side to digital communities. While my experience has been overwhelmingly positive, I have encountered some negativity and mean comments. An essay I wrote on acupuncture and holistic treatments was published on a widely read online platform that generated comments that ranged from critical and skeptical, to down-right mean. I stopped reading them and to this day will not revisit the comments board or even reread the essay. Another woman responded to a column I'd written about the benefits of herbal therapy with accusations of wrongdoing and anger; she couldn't accept that this was my experience and that I was sharing it with other sufferers.

How dare she give women false hope! This kind of stuff doesn't work—shame on her for touting it as a real solution.

While I took these messages to heart and often felt sick to my stomach over them, ultimately I received many more positive than negative messages which made sharing my experience worth it in the end. If my story can provide comfort or hope to other women out there, even if it's only just a few, it's totally worth it. I'd take all the mean, hateful comments for the loving, supportive, and encouraging ones. The women who reach out with their questions, stories, and tips have been invaluable. In this emotionally-draining and lonely endo-world, these women make me feel whole again.

There was the woman who reached out on Facebook and asked me questions about my holistic regime. She was interested in trying a more natural, alternative approach after her doctor was pushing her to go on Lupron after having the second laparoscopy that, at the time, she was preparing for. There was the woman who sent long, newsy letters of her own positive holistic experience and encouraged me to continue writing this book, who entered my life serendipitously at the exact moment that I thought I might give up writing about endo completely; There was the woman who emailed me from a dark, hopeless, painful place, who'd come across an essay I'd written about my success with different alternative treatments and suddenly felt like there could be another way, another path to healing after her own failed laparoscopies and Western treatments.

Then, of course there is comedy in pain. I belong to one group on Facebook that is devoted entirely to memes about endometriosis and women's health. Endo warriors post about heating pads, bloated bellies, bowel movements (I may be thirty-six, but poop jokes still make me laugh like a toddler). I appreciate having an audience to joke with about how I pee more frequently than an old man with a bad prostrate. Sometimes, laughing when it hurts can be just as healing as a castor oil pack or good cup of herbal tea.

17

BEAUTY IN PAIN: ART & CHRONIC ILLNESS

I never really understood abstract artwork until I experienced chronic physical pain. How can someone represent esoteric, enigmatic ideas in neat, pretty pictures? Love, pain, and grief are ineffable things—and if words can't capture the feelings behind them then how can images? My pain—my endometriosis—resembled a Jackson Pollack painting, its abstract lesions painted across the canvas of my organs in frenzied strokes. Language would be insufficient in conveying this kind of pain, but I would gravitate towards modernist renderings which seemed to offer a kind of preternatural understanding. During the worst of it, I recognized my body in the expressionist portraits of Egon Schiele, his renderings of the human form—twisted, contorted, grotesque, sensual, ugly —would strike me at my core. His work would force me to contemplate all the ways in which the ugliness of the human condition is also beautiful.

And I sought this clarity in other art forms. The unconventional poetry of Gertrude Stein—her strange interrogation of language and nature present in her repetition spoke to this pain and all the ways it distorts tradition. I modeled her style as I wrote through my chronic illness: *This is pain. This is a woman in pain. This is endometriosis. This is heartbreak, heartache, hearts aching and breaking and bodies aching and breaking. Endometriosis.*

Then there was music. Angry, aggressive heavy metal like Slipknot. Corey Taylor's voice ranged from guttural to melodic and even poetic, expressing frustration, rage, sadness—a perfect soundtrack for chronic pain. Sometimes, I wanted to scream but it felt just as good to listen to Corey Taylor do it (and it certainly sounded better!). Other times I played melancholy songs that were more instrumental and soothing, an antidote to difficult moods. Halsey's voice, such a contrast to Taylor's, calmed and relaxed me. Perhaps their songs brought me even greater comfort at times since they were so vocal about their own battle with endometriosis. There were many musicians and songs that played on repeat during flare ups and depressive periods. I believe music, perhaps even more than other art forms, was vital in my path to healing. And certainly crucial in the book writing process. I don't think I could have devoted the hundreds of hours of research, writing, rewriting, and revision to this memoir without an inspiring soundtrack.

I always felt that I was most productive in my writing, my art, when I was suffering. I have tried to mend a broken heart with a keyboard and cup of tea. I chip away at the pain—fingers rhythmic against keyboards. Writing is comfort, understanding, decompression. This is how I process life and all of its complications, how I make sense of the incomprehensible. My father cheated; I wrote. My first love broke my heart; I wrote. I cheated and broke my own heart; I wrote. Depression and anxiety made it hard to breathe; I exhaled pages. Endometriosis ravaged my insides; I wrote the pain away, or, at least, I distracted myself from it.

Artists channel hurt and illness and use it to fuel creation. Frida Kahlo was bed ridden and riddled with chronic pain; she created surrealist paintings. Virginia Woolf and Sylvia Plath suffered great mental anguish, and, before ending their lives, they wrote exquisite literary works.

In the 19th century, Charlotte Perkins Gilman wrote the short story *The Yellow Wallpaper* to criticize her mistreatment by the medical field of her day. Suffering from depression, she was prescribed a rest cure which didn't even allow her to pick up a pen to write. On the brink of complete mental breakdown, Gilman rejected her doctor and became her own advocate, returning to her writing and, in effect, saving herself from insanity. In the late 19th, early 20th century, women writers were not simply using their craft to endure chronic conditions, they were defying their patriarchal society by their acts of writing and publishing.

Perhaps this memoir is an act of defiance; I'm defying western medicine, society, and my own shortcomings. But writing about my pain, perhaps, is also a form of rehabilitation. Translating these difficult moments into prose and the act of finding the right language when no words exist to accurately capture the essence of the pain—the physical agony plus the mental anguish, the frustration, the hopelessness, the kind of pain that most people wouldn't understand—the pain that pushes a body to it's breaking point, to the point of vomiting, to shaking because it is so traumatic—is therapeutic in a way.

Transcribing pain onto the page has been transformative; it has allowed me to overcome my physical restrictions in a sense, like meditation or LSD (not that I've ever taken a hallucinogen!) I understand and come to terms with things better when I write about them. It is part of the way I process trauma. For example, I didn't fully process the trauma of sexual assault until I wrote an essay about it. Writing about pain allowed me to look at it from an objective perspective— to view it as something which didn't belong to me and only me, but rather, to many. It is not something which separates and isolates but something that unifies. Out of one, many. I've made connections to other women suffering from endometriosis and they have helped me in invaluable ways. It is embarrassing as hell to share intimate details, to be vulnerable with strangers and family alike. I don't like to talk about my period or how I cheated on my boyfriend in college or how I sometimes have ridiculous pain when I orgasm. But the act itself of writing these painful moments and memories and then sharing it with others has perhaps been the most beautiful and productive thing I have ever done.

18
CHRONIC: A CONCLUSION

Dear reader, fellow endo-warrior, chronic pain-sufferer, woman hurting in silence,

This book is for you. It isn't a cure. It isn't a magical solution for your chronic pain. But, maybe, just maybe, some of my suggestions and experiences will help you feel better. Maybe you will make lifestyle and dietary changes, pursue a new holistic path, and ultimately find relief. Maybe you already control your disease with Western Medicine, but you'll discover you aren't alone in your suffering. Maybe this is a story you can relate to, a story with experiences that are also your experiences. Maybe you'll feel understood. Seen. Heard. Validated.

This is not an indictment of Western Medicine entirely—I did have years of pain-free existence thanks to the initial birth control pills I took. The argument could also be made that perhaps the path

I ultimately took toward healing would not have been successful if I had not had the laparoscopy, and, certainly, I would have never had an answer as to what was causing my pain without the surgical procedure. But Western Medicine generally fails women in pain. Society fails women in pain. *A woman in pain is not normal.*

As I stated in the beginning, this book is not meant to attack Western medicine, but rather, expose its flaws. I am not a medical professional of any kind—simply a professional patient. I only know my experience and my experience is this: surgery did not help my endo other than to provide me with a diagnosis. I experienced relief and healing with Eastern medicine. I know most women who've had excision surgeries for endo typically have at least two or three. I haven't needed another one—yet. I have my life back. Yes, I have occasional nights when I'm awake, curled on the bathroom floor in pain but they are not a part of my normal routine any more. I can honestly say that I feel free, liberated. Of course, this doesn't mean I won't relapse. But as of the writing of this book, it has been six years of manageable pain and minimal disruption to my days.

I've learned that pain is a language, the body's way of communicating with you. It has nuance—varying tone, word choice, and, like with any relationship, in order to cultivate the healthiest relationship possible with your body, you simply need to pay attention to the details. Listen to the way your body hurts—intense cramping, radiating pain or sharp, stabbing bursts of agony? Does it come on sudden and overwhelming, a violent mood swing triggered by nothing—or does it creep up on you, slowly, gradually building? These are some of the questions we must ask our bodies, and it is up to us to hear the answers she gives. Doctors or naturopaths can serve as our mediators or relationship counselors or therapists, and they can help translate this intricate monologue, but ultimately it is up to us to do the work. However, unlike relationships with others, we don't have an option to separate or divorce. We cannot end amicably or contentiously; we cannot end it at all so we have no other choice but to succeed, to communicate, and to love. We must love this broken, battered, war-torn body that is ours simply because it is ours.

For a time, my body was not my own. It belonged to the lovers I took to boost my ego; it belonged to my ex-boyfriend whose possessiveness and adoration of it was something I savored, something I wished I could experience for myself; for a time, it was alcohol's, it was pills, it was the food I did and didn't eat, it was the pain that dominated it like the possessive ex I finally left. It was the body my father criticized as too fat, the body my mother praised as healthy, and the body I saw in the mirror as disgusting. It was the body I compared to other women's bodies—my two sisters' bodies that were petite and perfect; my friends' bodies that were athletic and beautiful and smaller than mine; the other college girls' bodies with their expensive clothes that flattered narrow waists, long, lean legs, and pronounced collar bones, these young Boston University women who, my freshmen year, were voted the hottest all-American girls by Maxim Magazine.

And now my body belongs to me. I am a thirty-six-year-old woman, a wife, a mother, a teacher, a writer, an endo-warrior. I have found a workout regime that is manageable as a working mom. I've cultivated healthy eating habits. I love my holistic rituals for the relief they give me, but also for the body that exists because of them. My body will never look like Instagram fitness models or pop stars or the stick-thin coeds who still populate my college memories. And that's completely okay.

This book is meant to offer you hope, comfort, a friend. Its purpose is to tell you that you aren't going through chronic illness all by yourself. Another woman out there understands the pain you've experienced and the many ways it impacts your life. This woman gets it. She understands your complicated relationship with your body because she has one too.

Deriving meaning from illness can be comforting. I've come to believe that endometriosis isn't my punishment, my curse, my albatross, or my arch nemesis. It doesn't get to have an identity because that would give it power. It is simply a part of me. It doesn't define me or control my life anymore. I'm free. I'm free because I manage it with my holistic methods. I'm free because I accept that it belongs to me as much as my love of long car rides with the windows down, playing loud music while cooking, and a good cup of tea. I'm free because I've turned my endometriosis into my inspiration. My story. My raison d'etre.

A woman in pain is not unusual. But, dear reader, let us never accept it as normal. Let our fight be the element of pain that remains chronic. Let us persist. Always.

Yours,
Rebecca

Appendix

1. Endometriosis.org. *Facts about Endometriosis – Endometriosis.org*, http://endometriosis.org/resources/articles/facts-about-endometriosis/

2. "Lupron: National Women's Health Network." *National Women's Health Network* |, 24 Dec. 2020, https://nwhn.org/tag/lupron/

3. Dubowsky, Jennifer. "Pulse Power: Understanding Pulses in Chinese Medicine." *Qi Blog*, 16 Oct. 2014, https://qiblog.emperors.edu/2014/09/pulse-power-understanding-tcm-pulse-diagnosis/

4. http://www.acupuncture.edu/2016/09/28/understanding-tongue-diagnosis-in-chinese-medicine/

5. *Define_me*, https://www.fertstert.org/article/S0015-0282(10)00980-5/pdf#:~:text=In%201903%2C%20Mayer%20(14),glands%20around%20the%20silk%20ligatures

6. Pcom. "TCM to Treat Endometriosis Symptoms." *Pacific College*, 8 Jan. 2019, https://www.pacificcollege.edu/news/blog/2015/02/26/tcm-to-treat-endometriosis-symptoms

7. Cynthia Sass, MPH. "Matcha: Benefits, Nutrition, and Risks." *Health*, Health, 20 Sept. 2022, https://www.health.com/nutrition/what-is-matcha

8. Goodson, Amy. "Red Raspberry Leaf Tea: Pregnancy, Benefits and Side Effects." *Healthline*, Healthline Media, 30 July 2018, https://www.healthline.com/nutrition/red-raspberry-leaf-tea#benefits

9. "Avoiding Cold Beverages – Why?" *Nis Chinese Medical Center*, https://www.drboni.com/?p=496

10. "Endometriosis – A Chinese Medicine Approach." *The Yinova Center*, 28 Sept. 2021, https://www.yinovacenter.com/blog/endometriosis-a-chinese-medicine-approach/

11. "Spirulina: Dosage, Eye Health, Oral Health, and More." *Medical News Today*, MediLexicon International, https://www.medicalnewstoday.com/articles/324027.php

[12] "Health Concerns Cramp Bark plus - 90 Capsules." *Lhasa OMS*, https://www.lhasaoms.com/health-concerns-cramp-bark-plus

[13] Pcom. "TCM to Treat Endometriosis Symptoms." *Pacific College*, 8 Jan. 2019, https://www.pacificcollege.edu/news/blog/2015/02/26/tcm-to-treat-endometriosis-symptoms

[14] Kubala, Jillian. "Castor Oil: 4 Benefits and Uses." *Healthline*, Healthline Media,28 Jan. 2022, https://www.healthline.com/nutrition/castor-oil #TOC_TITLE_HDR_5

[15] Timmons, Jessica. "4 Best CBD Products for Endometriosis Pain 2022." *Healthline*, Healthline Media, 14 July 2022, https://www.healthline.com/ health/cbd-for-endometriosis#endocannabinoid-system

[16] Pcom. "TCM to Treat Endometriosis Symptoms." *Pacific College*, 8 Jan. 2019, https://www.pacificcollege.edu/news/blog/2015/02/26/tcm-to-treat-endometriosis-symptoms

[17] "Endometriosis – A Chinese Medicine Approach." *The Yinova Center*, 28 Sept. 2021, https://www.yinovacenter.com/blog/endometriosis-a-chinese-medicine-approach/

[18] Link, Rachael. "Dandelion: Health Benefits and Side Effects." *Healthline*, Healthline Media, 4 Jan. 2022, https://www.healthline.com/nutrition/ dandelion-benefits#TOC_TITLE_HDR_8

[19] "Milk Thistle." *National Center for Complementary and Integrative Health*, U.S. Department of Health and Human Services, https://nccih.nih.gov/ health/milkthistle/ataglance.htm

[20] Cook, Andrew S., and Danielle Cook. *The Endometriosis Health & Diet Program: Get Your Life Back*. Robert Rose Inc., 2017

[21] Xu, Juna. "50% Of Endometriosis Sufferers Have Suicidal Thoughts, New Study Finds." *Body and Soul*, 8 Oct. 2019, https://www.bodyandsoul.com.au/health/womens-health/50-of-endometriosis-sufferers-have-suicidal-thoughts-new-study-finds/news-story/ ff57e5bfd7c88e60751ba2a136442af8

[22] "How Ohnut Works." *OhnutCo*, https://ohnut.co/pages/how-it-works

[23] Betjes, Erik. "What Is Pelvic Floor Physical Therapy?" *ISSM*, 16 Dec. 2013, https://www.issm.info/sexual-health-qa/what-is-pelvic-floor-physical-therapy/

[24] "Could Pelvic Floor Physical Therapy Help You? - Health & Wellness." *Loma Linda University Health*, https://lluh.org/patients-visitors/health-wellness/could-pelvic-floor-physical-therapy-help-you

[25] "Natural Cycles Birth Control: No Hormones or Side Effects." *Natural Cycles*, 20 Oct. 2022, https://www.naturalcycles.com/

[26] Alighieri, Dante, and Allen Mandelbaum. *The Divine Comedy of Dante Alighieri, Inferno: A Verse Translation, with an Introduction by Allen Mandelbaum*. Bantam Books, 1988

[27] Bulletti, Carlo, et al. "Endometriosis and Infertility." *Journal of Assisted Reproduction and Genetics*, Springer US, Aug. 2010, https://www.ncbi.nlm.nih.gov/pmc/articles/PMC2941592/#:~:text=Endometriosis%20is%20a%20very%20common,endometriosis%20are%20infertile%20%5B4%5D

[28] Parenthood, Planned. "Birth Control Pills: The Pill: Contraceptive Pills." *Planned Parenthood*, https://www.plannedparenthood.org/learn/birth-control/birth-control-pill

[29] Cohut, Maria. "Female Hysteria: The History of a Controversial 'Condition.'" *Medical News Today*, MediLexicon International, 13 Oct. 2020, https://www.medicalnewstoday.com/articles/the-controversy-of-female-hysteria#Vibrators-for-hysteria?

[30] Villines, Zawn. "Is Endometriosis Hereditary? Research and Statistics." *Medical News Today*, MediLexicon International, 12 Feb. 2020, https://www.medicalnewstoday.com/articles/is-endometriosis-hereditary#is-it-hereditary

[31] Kelley, Geri. "Researchers to Study Possible Link between COVID-19 and Menstrual Changes." *MSU Today*, 30 Aug. 2021, https://msutoday.msu.edu/news/2021/researchers-to-study-possible-link-between-covid-19-and-menstrual-changes

[32] Muhaidat, Nadia, et al. "Menstrual Abnormalities after COVID-19 Vaccine: IJWH." *International Journal of Women's Health*, Dove Press, 28 Mar. 2022, https://www.dovepress.com/menstrual-symptoms-after-covid-19-vaccine-a-cross-sectional-investigat-peer-reviewed-fulltext-article-IJWH

Additional Resources

This treatment plan can function like a grab-bag of holistic treatments. It is comprehensive, curative, and customizable for each warrior.

SAMPLE DAILY ROUTINE:
Morning:
Before breakfast, take 6 Spirulina tablets, and a tablespoon of extra virgin olive oil. This is followed by a hot cup of lemon water then a cup of Matcha green tea.
Afternoon:
Drink two cups of Raspberry leaf or comparable herbal tea
Evening:
Drink hot water with dinner
Apply castor oil pack (3 times a week)
Drink milk thistle with water before bed

ESSENTIAL OILS
Castor oil
Extra virgin olive oil
Apple cider vinegar
Blackstrap Molasses
CBD Oil
evening primrose oil
clary sage
frankincense
 lavender
neroli
ylang ylang

TEAS
Raspberry Leaf
Mint teas—Spearmint and peppermint
Matcha Green tea
Dandelion
Turmeric

HERBS/SUPPLEMENTS
Spirulina
Maca root
Cramp Bark Plus
Vitamin B6
Vitamin D
Milk Thistle
Zinc

DIET
Gluten-free
Dairy-free
Coconut milk or oat milk substitutes
Avoid red meats
Consume hot, cooked foods and beverages
The Endometriosis Health & Diet Program by Dr. Andrew S. Cook and Danielle Cook.
The Four-Week Endometriosis Diet Plan by Katie Edmonds.
Whole New You: How Real Food Transforms Your Life, for a Healthier, More Gorgeous You: A Cookbook by Jessica Porter and Tia Mowry.

ALTERNATIVE PRACTICES & PRODUCTS FOR PAIN MANAGEMENT

Acupuncture
Massage Therapy
Osteopathic manipulative treatment
TENS machine
Yoga
Cryotherapy
Castor oil packs/heating pads

SEX & INTIMACY

Ohnut—This wearable customizes penetration depth and helps some women find physical relief during intercourse.
https://ohnut.co/products/ohnut-buffer-rings
NeuEve—hormone free, estrogen-free, gluten-free, soy-free, preservative-free, GMO-free natural vaginal moisturizers.
Natural Cycles Birth Control App—hormone-free, FDA cleared birth control app.
Pelvic Floor Therapy

RESOURCES FOR ADDITIONAL SUPPORT

Naturopathy –finding the right Naturopath to help customize a holistic treatment plan can be a vital service for those who suffer or suspect they suffer from endometriosis or other chronic pain.

Endometriosis.net—online community that offers support and resources including a weekly newsletter which provides the latest news in endometriosis research and treatment as well as opportunities to participate in clinical trials and research.

Endometriosis Foundation of America—Nonprofit organization dedicated to advocacy, research, and promoting education. Visit https://

www.endofound.org/ for resources, articles, events, and to purchase endometriosis merchandise (proceeds raise money for endo research).

The Future Family—concierge fertility specialists offering services for women suffering from infertility-related endometriosis.

Pacific College.edu/news/endometriosis—offers additional information about Eastern Medicine's approach to endometriosis

Dr. Lj Endometriosis Coach & Wholistic Endo Expert— Functional Medicine + Strategy + Systems to empower, educate and motivate EndoWarriors to kick pain, fatigue and bloating. Dr. Lj offers self-paced courses, a podcast, blog, coaching service, and vibrant online community, you can find it all at https://www.ljspowerhouse.org/. You can also follow her on Instagram @ljs_powerhouse.

Tik Tok for Endo Awareness—A surprising place to find support, creators on this social media platform such as Sarah @kissmeormissme, Bloody Honest @bloodyhonest, Endometriosis Awareness @endobattle, Josie @josephinedbarr, Abbie @cheerfullylive, and Ashleigh Thiel @ashleight819 offer entertaining, humorous, creative content for endo-warriors.

Acknowledgments

I want to thank David LeGere and Christopher Madden for believing in this book. You have both supported and encouraged me more than you know, and I am eternally grateful.

Thank you Sonya Huber for giving me the courage to write the book that needed to be written.

Thank you Jennifer Dimyan and Don Quaintance for inspiring me to try something new.

Thank you to the women who read my articles and essays, who reached out with your own stories and questions and fears and frustrations. This book wouldn't exist without you.

Thank you to all my friends and family. You are my everything.

And finally, I want to thank Greg, the hero of my story yesterday, today, and forever.

About the Author

Rebecca Dimyan is an award-winning writer, editor, and teacher. Her work has been published in national and international publications including *Vox*, the *CT Post, YahooHealth, 34th Parallel, Glassworks Magazine, The Mighty* and many others. She has taught college writing at several universities in Connecticut for nearly a decade. Rebecca is also an experienced editor and conference director. Her debut novel *Waiting for Beirut* was a finalist for the 2021 Fairfield Book Prize. Rebecca's book *Chronic: A Memoir of Illness & Healing* delves into her experience with chronic illness and alternative medicine.